Life

Is A

Shared Creation

Life is A Shared Creation

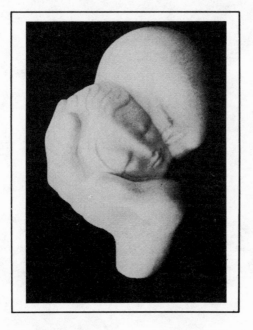

by

Paul Brenner, M.D.

DeVorss & Company, Publishers
P. O. Box 550
Marina del Rey, California 90291

First paperback edition 1981
Second printing October 1981

ISBN No. 0-87516-454-4

Stone Sculpture
Titled: *A Shared Creation*
by
Dean Mars
Santa Barbara, CA

I would like to acknowledge all people, all things and all of life's processes in the writing of this book. *Life is A Shared Creation* represents my personal attempt to tap and record this evolving Collective Creative Consciousness.

Life is A Shared Creation is my gift to its creator, *All*.

Table of Contents

POSTPARTUM

Preface

Life is conceived in a thought that gives birth to a form. That initial intent to give life to life is what perpetuates life itself. As creative beings, each moment of our lives is pregnant and as such has the potential to be life everlasting. *Life is A Shared Creation* speaks to that creatively evolving, transformational process. In the pages that follow, life is viewed through the transparency of birth and parenthood.

Life is A Shared Creation is written to challenge some of the myths of birth and to make couples more aware of the responsibility that parenthood carries. At the same time, this book attempts to explain how a child is an active participant in his or her own creation. Therefore, this book is not written solely for those who are anticipating childbirth, but it is written for all of us who once were children. The Book explains how we, as a people, are interconnected with one another and with our past.

The book speaks metaphorically to the birth of any creative endeavor. *Life is A Shared Creation* is written for All and belongs to All.

My sincere hope is that you, the reader, may touch the love that is found within your own essence and so accept that same spark of creation within others. My hope also is that you may be moved as a result of this insight to contact your family and friends by either a letter, a call, a hug, or a pregnant moment of silent thought to give rebirth to that *Love,* the source of *All* creation.

Life is a Shared Creation

Divine Love
fills and covers your being.
Go forth into the world
for you have received
the breath of
God.

Your gift of life
is to share
in the universal force of
Love.

Your gift to life
is to manifest
your divinity,
to see that same
Light
in all others and all things,
to transform that
Energy
into works of
Love
and so
to make visible
The Collective Creative Consciousness.

Your Essence is
God.
Your purpose
is to evolve
God.
Your Gift to Life is A Shared Creation
with
ALL.

I

Love is the translucent thread that runs through creation, life, and healing

The Introduction

Autobiography • Illness • Health
Love • Life • Creation

I n 1933 I was born the fourth child into the family of Anne and Isadore
Brenner. Their first child, a son, died in childbirth. My early
life was filled with not only the love of my parents but that
of my sisters, Sybil and Claire. Those years were also laced
with moments of violent outbursts by my father. His frustration stemmed from an unfulfilled desire to be a physician. Being the youngest child of immigrants, he was forced
to leave school at age 11 to help finance his oldest brother's
education in law. His family's dream was that one member
of the Brenner brood of 1900 would make it over the ghetto
wall.

It now becomes understandable why, following the acci-
dental death of my closest friend when I was 10 years old,
my father responded to my emotional crying need to prevent death, to be a doctor. Through personal family sacrifice, I was soon launched on a twenty-year educational
odyssey that included the Hotchkiss School, Brown University, New York Medical College, general internship,
residency training in obstetrics and gynecology, sub-
specialty training in female cancer surgery, and finally,
what I thought was the ultimate double golden ring
ceremony of the medical marriage: a teaching position at
the University of California School of Medicine at San
Diego, and a private practice. My education was a narrow,
straight-ahead pattern through the science of medicine during the Golden Age of Technology. My medical career was

3

integrated with my marriage to Joyce and the birth of our family; Bradford, Elisabeth and Ilene.

My life, however, began to change when, in 1972, I was introduced to acupuncture. This most ancient oriental art of healing, at first glance, seemed ridiculous. How could needles placed in various skin areas effect medical cures? How could the Chinese possibly feel that there were methods to regulate energy flow throughout the body? What energy? But, on second glance, it worked. Acupuncture, which still defies all scientific paradigms, led me to further my studies in alternative forms of healing such as hypnosis, faith healing, and American Indian medicine. I was drawn to study Zen, Taoism, and the Kabala and, in time, realized the similarity between religion, philosophy, and science. However, it was not until 1976, when I took a leave of absence from obstetrics and gynecology to counsel the chronically ill, that I learned that conception, pregnancy, and childbirth are, respectively, methaphors for love, life, and creation.

I felt compelled to leave traditional medicine to explore further those factors related to health and illness. Up until the present writing, I have limited my new practice to one patient per day. The entire day, if necessary, is devoted to that person. I no longer am restricted by a full waiting room or the pressures of an impending surgery or delivery. This format heightens my awareness of those personal yet human factors that might be related to the appreciation of life or to its absence—illness. These singular open-ended counseling sessions (which are held in my home or garden) allow ample time for the patients to present their entire autobiographies.

During that unobstructed period, at times six to eight hours, each person becomes more than a patient. That person becomes a friend. Paradoxically, each friend also becomes a healer who, during our mutual interactions, often heals deep, forgotten wounds within me. Each has taught me the meaning of the wounded healer, that the ill are an untapped natural resource to teach health to the healthy. These most patient friends and teachers are my

mirrors, and I now understand more of the interconnectedness that links all humankind. I realize that the patient-
doctor relationship is a reciprocal one in which both are
simultaneously serving each other.

As these people shared their life stories, I saw myself.
Their parents, their families, their loves, and their pains
were similar and, at times, identical in content to my own.
The major portion of each session was devoted to unravel-
ing and then resolving the client's unfinished business with
his or her close personal relations. I soon understood illness
to be a forceful reminder (in a sense, a friend) that prods us
to reassess the meaning of life.

Most of the people I saw happened to have chronic illness
or cancer. The individual who has been labeled "terminal"
usually communicates more freely about his or her innermost joys, fears, loves, and sorrows. They remind me of
Janis Joplin when she sang Kris Kristofferson's lines,
"Freedom's just another word for nothin' else to lose." The
dying often brought me back to the stage of life called birth.

I met young cancer patients in their twenties and thirties
whose birth and formative years were enveloped in a
chaotic family environment and who, at an early age, had
already begun to reenact their parents' scenarios. I met
numerous older persons who still carried the frustration and
anger of their parents' disharmonious relationships, especially when those intimate personal bonds were shrouded in
unresolved conflict.

I realized how these familiar yet unpleasant situations are
dutifully repeated generation after generation until a solution is found in understanding and/or in love. In such a manner, we create our own universe of learning experiences and
resolutions. The resolution of personal conflict with close
family members seems to be a needed step for either the living of life or the acceptance of death. Therefore, if the
understanding of this human process can be appreciated
before and after conception, then the chronic suffering of
humankind may be replaced by acute periods of tolerable
discomfort.

I am reminded of a 68-year old woman who was dying

from a cancer diagnosed as being untreatable. When I first met her, she was frail and could hardly breathe to speak. When she did speak, she spoke only in anger about her mother, who had died thirty years before but who, she felt, was the cause of her unhappy marriage and illness. She blurted, "I was not wanted from birth!" However, one day, while sitting in my back yard, she recalled an incident when, as a teenager, she broke up with her first love. She remembered sitting on a stool in the kitchen, crying uncontrollably. She then described how her mother entered the room and quietly placed a hand on her head and said, "Mein Kind, mein Kind—it will be all right—it will be all right." In that moment of recall, the woman screamed, "My God, she loved me! She loved me!" The joy filling her heart still lingers throughout the gardens of my back yard. In that moment of understanding and acceptance, she took her first breath for life, for rebirth. With that breath, the pain of cancer disappeared. The void created by the absence of pain was replaced by the inspiration of love.

Following that momentous day for both of us, she began to awaken as early as 5:30 in the morning to walk the magnificent deserted beaches with her husband. She later told me, "Paul, I never lived a day in my life until I had cancer. Through cancer, I found my mother—I found myself." I remember well both my astonishment and my silence. She continued, "Although I have lived in San Diego for over thirty years, I never purposely watched a sunset or even reflected for but a moment upon the wonderment of my own existence—I was too busy. But following the diagnosis of my cancer and my acceptance of my mother and her love, I now awake early in the morning and walk the beaches with my husband. I now cherish each day and each moment I share with my family, my friends and perhaps more importantly with myself. I now relish the quietness of my own solitude. I have become spellbound, mesmerized, by the fall sunsets and find myself softly acknowledging how blessed I am to have experienced life. I am aware of a new voice from within which, during these incredible moments, whispers, 'Thanks.'" She continued, "What if I had been killed on the freeway or had suffered a fatal heart attack and had never experienced these past few months?"

Six months after this most memorable day, my friend was dead. But I feel she died in health. For me, health now means the appreciation and acceptance of life. As of this date, I have not met a single cancer person who, after deep soul searching, has not confided to me that cancer was the most significant turning point in their life. For these people, cancer was not only physically transforming, but spiritually transforming. Health is the acceptance of life, not necessarily the condition of one's body. These people made me aware that most of us plod blindly through life unthinking, asleep, yet unconsciously seeking some shock that will awaken us to the full realization of our being. All too often that shock, that stimulus, comes in the form of illness.

These "ill people" became my teachers and posed endless questions to me: Do I need cancer, a heart attack, or for that matter, any illness to make today count? Do I need to catch my thumb in a door to appreciate my hand? Or can I consciously merge with the sun, the beaches, the oceans, the mountains, the deserts, and most importantly, with myself and those whom I love, with those whom I touch and those who touch me? Why cannot all of this take place in times of health? Can I learn to accept and love myself without the need for illness?

The most worthwhile counseling sessions often left me in a state of confusion as to who was the "client" and who was the "therapist," who was the student, and who was the teacher. More frequently than not, the sessions extended an additional hour as I shared with the "client" what I, the "therapist," had learned. They, in turn, shared their newly found insights with me. This was often followed by another half hour as we embraced at the door, both about to burst with love, knowing, and tears of joy.

My friends taught me love. They taught me that if I block or shield myself from love, I am setting the stage for uncontrolled stress: distress. If I am afraid to allow myself to experience love, my beingness contracts and converts my essence from a fluid state to a solid one. I became aware that it is this contracted state that is illness. They also taught me that if I allow love in and then try to hold on to it, possess it, that this attachment will limit me from experiencing myself and others. Finally, they taught me UN-CONDITIONAL LOVE, love based on the total acceptance of life and life's conditions. It is hoped in the future it will be this type of love that prompts us to create, to share, to bear children.

I could not help but learn how the parents' intentions before pregnancy, the interpersonal relationships of parents during their pregnancy, the events of delivery, and the ambiance of those first years of life help mold the child and shape the health of the adult. I have been guided through the full cycle of life by the chronically ill and dying as they have led me back to obstetrics, the field of medicine dealing with the creation of life. But this time I return with a deeper understanding of that life energy, and a need to share, through this book, the wisdom that often comes through illness. Perhaps, someday, we will be able to learn without suffering and without disease. The teacher will be love.

To begin, first one must begin at the beginning. Conception, pregnancy, delivery, and the post-partum period are to me the most appropriate moments to establish the milieu for future physical, mental, and spiritual health. These most memorable and, yes, momentous events cannot be taken lightly. The newborn is a totally receptive being who is the role model for unconditional love. The babe is a being who does not discern, but accepts whatever his or her parents or the environment offers.

Life is conceived as a thought, a thought in the parents' minds before conception, and often continues beyond the delivery into that child's adulthood. That new life, as a fine wine that was conceived in the mind of the vintner, still has a variable gestation period depending on the uniqueness of his or her essence. In a similar manner, like life, the completion of the aged wine is only in its sharing. The true pregnancy is not completed until the child becomes an active participant, a co-creator, in the collectively shared experience called life. Birth, like life, is not easy. Birth makes its demands, as does life, and out of these demands gives birth to its rewards and so to evolving life.

Thus, the moment heralding conception bonds the parent and child for eternity. Though inseparable, as the sculptor and the stone, each participant must maintain his or her own integrity, his or her own uniqueness. This is the paradox that exists between the creator and those things created, between the energy of thought and the energy of form. It is all the same, yet it is different. These eternal bonds of co-creation between mother, father and child exist whether the conceptus is aborted, a stillborn or survives a half-century or more with its creator. The quality of a lifetime cannot be judged or qualified by our limited sense of relative time. In truth, parenthood and life precede conception, while pregnancy continues beyond birth. It is for this reason that pregnancy affords us a unique model by which we can analyze the creator and the creation over both a relative and absolute lifetime. Birth is a metaphor for that life spiral and that needed love.

In the beginning there was thought. The initial thought to sustain humanity was love. That thought continues still and forever into eternity. Love remains the only word worth conceiving, worth sharing.

The thought of love is the bond, the translucent thread that runs through all teachings about creation and life, linking the myriad projections, sensations, and emotions which fill the time span from the first intention to conceive, to the birth, or even death, of that intention. Once the perfection of this thread is recognized and followed, it becomes strong enough to sustain together the husband and wife, the mother and father, and that jewel in the necklace, the newborn.

Love, as well as the genetic code, has the power to be transmitted through each dividing cell of the unfolding embryo. This love can serve as a template for the quality of life for your child and the quality of love for generations to come. CONCEPTION is a gift of love, PREGNANCY is a gift to life, and LIFE is a shared creation for all.

Thus, life can be told through the story of birth and

parenthood. The formless thought of love gives birth to a form called a human being. That formed soul, conceived in love, now enters a state of moment to moment births and deaths called life. Each moment of life so becomes pregnant for that unique soul and each cycle is strung upon the thread of love as a continuum of pearls called the life process. Each new rebirth offers a gift to life which can now be shared by all of its members called humanity. These gifts which were created from the source of all love are now delivered in love by that soul as an offering of life to life.

This infinitely evolving thread of a Transforming Absolute Love is called A Shared Creation.

II | *Thought is the seed for eternal transformation.*

The Power of Thought

Energy • Transformation • Thought
Love • Conscious Conception

Pregnancy begins prior to conception as an act of creative thought. That thought has a lifetime of its own and thereby continues to shape the form it conceived. The parental thought to conceive or not to conceive is analogous to the sculptor's choice of stone or medium to be sculpted. A sculptor surveys the entire stone before surrendering the chisel to the force of the mallet. Each surface is carefully inspected. Its faults are consciously analyzed. The stone selected dictates the feasibility of carrying out the artist's projections and so the stone is a co-creator in its final form. The stone essentially speaks to the sculptor, stating clearly what can be accomplished. A mental survey precedes the moment when human force meets resistant stone. The moment the chisel is set to the stone, the thought begins its journey through the life of that unique stone. Until that time, all is conjecture.

All life's creations involve the transformation of a singular formless thought of love into a multitude of manifest loves. It is through such a transformational process that humankind infinitely evolves, infinitely aspires, and so, once again, returns to Absolute Love. All our formed endeavors, be they our children or our work, are but gifts that are offered to life for the privilege of being. The more clearly we transform that formless love, the closer our gifts represent the source from which they came. This book represents the duality of form and formless that merge in the creation of life itself.

The time-honored dilemma of which comes first, the chicken or the egg, appears unanswerable. Life and creation are inseparable. Each moment of our lives is involved in a creative process, whether walking, talking, writing, or making love, but pregnancy is the most explicit biological example of this simultaneous fusion of the creator and the creation. Perhaps a more profound thought would be: What precedes the chicken and the egg?

If, as modern physics dictates in the first law of thermodynamics, energy cannot be created or destroyed, then the question must be posed: Are we humans capable of creating or destroying anything? Are we but one form of life energy that interacts with but another form of the same energy to produce a new variant? Does the energy of the child exist prior to conception, and does the new creation, the newborn, represent recycled energy that can only be reshaped by life's circumstances? Is birth preceded by a type of transitory death of all its participants? Does modern science validate the ancient religious belief of the eternal individual soul and the universal energy of spirit? If physics is correct, then is the child an active participant with both universal energy and with its parents in birth? Do we mere humans behave as particles of energy? Even if not, can we transpose some of the wisdom of physics into our own lives?

If we can accept this continuum of living energy as a possible truth for but a moment, then we cannot help but be more accepting of each individual life and that life's experience as being essential for the evolution of both that individual and the collective energy of all humankind. It would also mean that we are not only living out our own lives, but at the same time, through interpersonal transactions, we are living through the lives of our fellow humans and, in turn, our lives are lived through theirs. This realization should logically diminish our need either to compare or judge one life or its purpose with another and to diminish the self-destructive acts of war and hate.

If, indeed, energy cannot be created or destroyed, then all life is based on a given quantity of energy. Humankind's destiny is to change the quality of that life within a system of defined energy. Therefore, the parents and the child become co-creators in an evolving quality of human consciousness and the form it takes. My premise is that *CO-CREATION IS NOT A CREATIVE PROCESS, BUT A TRANSFORMATIONAL ONE.* Energy is always there. We cannot create energy, but we can mold energy to bring form out of the formless and, so to speak, make love. Transformation is the only means for humankind to elevate love to an even higher plane. The converse is also true, for we only transform through love. Co-creation is essential for the *quality* of an evolving human consciousness, and thus evolution is born out of the transformation of disparate sources of the same energy. For the human being, evolution is dependent upon the unique differences offered by its participants. In the case of our total human existence, evolution is dependent upon the interactions of various people, religions, and nations. The outcome of all these labored human relationships reflects the quality of love that we have made available to the generations that are to follow. The child in a very real sense is love made visible.

So life, as told through the story of pregnancy, conception—creation—occurs not only in the moment when the sperm penetrates the egg, but when the ripe energy of parental thought fuses with the unblemished energy of the yet unborn; then the newborn and the new father and new mother, the new wife and the new husband, are the new qualitative bursts of renascent energy that have taken form in the fusion of variable energies. However, newness demands the surrender of what was. In a very real sense, life begins before conception, is reshaped by birth, and exists beyond death.

Since thought usually precedes action, a decision to enter into the birth process, or any other creative endeavor, should be based on an in-depth analysis of the content in that thought. A three-dimensional analysis of our thoughts to conceive (*why* do I want a child, when do I want a child, and if I do indeed conceive, how will my life be affected) should lead to either a more conscious pregnancy or a more conscious form of birth control. For those who *consciously* choose the former, the birth itself will more likely be welcomed with a joyous celebration, which wraps the child in love for a lifetime or longer. Thoughts, too, have a life process of their own. Thoughts are not planar but can be scrutinized in depth. If we recognize that the child's nourishment begins with the initial intent, and not with conception, then thoughts are equivalent to a contract that must be honored.

Even after such soul searching, life still offers choices and probabilities—not guarantees. As the barker at the fair warns, "Pay ya money—and take ya choice." Therefore, preconception is a time not only to reflect on personal thoughts and feelings, but to renew marital contracts. Honest, open communication, stated in a nonjudgmental, nonthreatening atmosphere can strengthen any marriage and lay a firm foundation for the future family. If the decision is to conceive a child, then the relative harmony or disharmony created through your shared choice can affect the quality of the child's life. Your decision is equivalent to the consummation of the act of creation.

The outcome of every conception is an unknown. If a couple is willing to accept this contractual risk, then there is no other option but to accept the choice unconditionally. From the birth of the child on, life itself will present its own conditions for growth and transformation. How both the parents and the child respond to life's conditions will be reflected in the participant's relative happiness, joy, pain, or sorrow.

And so it follows that thought and the power of its initial stimulus shapes form. Thought is the seed of probability and probability is the seed of creation. The only absolute is the Absolute. Fortunately, unlike the sculptor's chisel, thought is not set in stone. If thought can create form, then thought can mold pre-existing form. It is never too late to create a new thought form or change an old one. Like gamma rays and x-rays, thought is another aspect of universal energy; it, too, is transmutable. But this often escapes our attention because it is not within our ordinary visual field and cannot be contained in a box.

There is more than what can be seen, felt or determined genetically that is transmittable. This is well documented by behavioral researchers who demonstrate similar behavioral patterns between twins that have been separated and reared independently. They often demonstrate identical preferences for clothes, food, or even type of spouse. There are also interesting behavioral patterns that have been reported between adopted children and their biologic parents. Often these children share common hobbies and professions of their biologic parents. Is inheritance behavioral? Is inheritance genetic? Or more likely is it a combination of both?

More recently as a result of research with recombinant DNA techniques, scientists have found that genes can flip over, shuffle and pop in and out of what were once thought to be immutable positions. At present the answer to what the prime mover is for "jumping genes" is unknown. I, therefore, feel free to fill the void of this unknown with a personal hypothesis, and that is that thought shapes form and that our consciousness causes genes "to jump," to shift, and to dance out not only our inheritance but our health as well as our illness. We are the center and the cause of our personal reality.

Pregnancy is the time to expand the Cartesian dictum, "I think, therefore I am," to "I *think, therefore I transform.*" Thought may not replace the importance of the genetic pool nor affect the randomness of it, but thought can affect the quality of a child's existence. The newborn is not only a bond between the husband and wife, created through a mutual biologic communion, but in another sense, the newborn may be an energy field magnetized by a parental thought field. The author, Ray Bradbury, once said, "We are matter and form making itself over into imagination and will!"

A powerfully directed formless thought (will power) can penetrate and fertilize the formed cell with the same fervor as the relentless undulating sperm that dares to pierce the resistant radiant crown of the female egg. The fertilized cell, like the wave and particle components of light, represents both idea-like and matter-like characteristics. The initial thought to conceive, to transform life, is an act of both insemination and fertilization. To will means to invest in future probabilities and not in absolutes. But it *must* be understood that the thoughts that fill our intentions are our personal statements and investments in the quality of life.

So we see that thought can affect our children perhaps as inalterably and as dramatically as the genetic code dictates their physical form. All parents, even surrogate mothers (those who have volunteered to bear the child after being artificially inseminated by the husband of a sterile wife), as well as those who are considering giving up children for adoption, can have thoughts which continue to affect their shared child through its life. There is no distance too far or object too dense to prevent the reception or penetration of a singularly held projection. Individuals, even though separated by space, can be in constant communication, and through thoughts of love can continue to nurture their child. Either fear of separation or its opposite, the desire for freedom, are paradoxical illusions created through self-centeredness. We cohabit space and time and, therefore, are inseparably free.

At the same time, it is self-injustice for parents to torture themselves with lifelong guilt for actions or thoughts which may have brought their child unhappiness or illness. Some parents even feel inadequate because their baby was conceived by artificial insemination or surrendered to adoption. To compare oneself to another or to any illusion of the so-called norm is to be stuck in the guilt of the past and to miss the mark of the present. We can do no more than accept the results of our choices without judgment and then get on with living. With the acceptance of ourselves and our humanness, we are also preparing ourselves to cherish that new entering life energy, no matter what form or experience of life either our sons or our daughters choose.

Much has been written in the last ten years about how people are totally responsible for all the situations in life in which they find themselves, either physically or mentally. Response and responsibility come from the root Latin word *respondere*—to reply. Our choices in life, our replies, are what define the stimuli of our life. "The Devil made me do it!" The question is: Who did it? Who defined the stimulus? If you are given a rose for the first time, it will be defined by your responses. This may take the form of joy from its scent, pain from its thorns, or a combination of both. The circumstances of our birth and our experiences in life may be emotionally beyond our control but, more importantly, how have they moved us to our present condition? Which option did we personally choose in response to a given situation? What alternatives did we bypass?

Responsibility does not mean blame or connote guilt, but responsibility does demand a personal response to the conditions of life that prod us into action. The author-philosopher Hermann Hesse stated it simply: "I hold that I am not responsible for the meaningfulness or the meaninglessness of my life, but I am responsible for what I do with my unique life."

I am reminded of writing my son a note after he left college to be a rock guitarist. "Dear Brad, I just want you to know I love you, whatever you do." He interpreted the letter to mean, "Even though I screw up, you'll love me." I held one intention, yet he had the option to choose another. The direction he took was, "I'll show you what I can do!" In the future, I may be judged as the spark for either Bradford's failure or success, but in the final analysis, my son is responsible for his own choices, his own gifts to life.

I must also admit that I remember the week that my son was conceived. I was in my second year of medical school and studying for the medical National Boards. I remember praying to God that if Joyce and I had children, that at least one would be so bright, so facile at school that either he or she would never be sitting in panic over a stack of books as I was at that moment and had been for most of my life. I also distinctly remember adding an addendum to my prayer. I prayed that that child would be a musician, a being who could share its life's vocation with others and at the same time use the same gift for self-enjoyment, a child whose hobby would be his life's work. I received my wish (Bradford) but my wish also has a life process of his own. I wish my wish well. The children that followed, Elisabeth and Ilene, were perhaps blessed by not being blessed by a paternal projection of the moment.

Creation takes place through interaction. Even in parthenogenesis, which is the development of an egg without fertilization, the stimulus which is necessary to trigger this process becomes the co-creator in the egg. The duality of opposite or variant forces is needed to give energy to either thought, form, or movement. Creation is the metaphor for comprehending life's paradox of duality and yet, prophetically, paradox is the parent of creation. The quality of both our love and maturity can be judged by the degree to which we accept the creations that are born from paradox or crisis. So beware of prolonged bliss; it may be a sign that you are either stuck, unstimulated, out of balance or even infertile.

Paradox is resolved in that instant of stillness when the pendulum that swings through all the combinations and permutations of life's variables is balanced at centerpoint. The moment of truth is when the centerpost comes in balance with the crossbar. This moment is also the point when unity is found in diversity. During this stillpoint in time, night is absorbed into day, death into life, and illness into health. But as the pendulum meets the resistance of its past, a new arc, a new spiral is created. Therefore, paradox, the horns of the dilemma, in the moment of resolution not only gives birth to the unicorn but also to a new set of paradoxes, to a new set of unknowns, which demands a new set of solutions. The simultaneous resolution and evolution of paradox is the weight of the cross and the joy of the transformational process. Life is not problems, Life is solutions.

Balance is life's struggle yet life's grace. Thus, there are new nights, new deaths, new illnesses to be counterbalanced by new days, new births, and new health. Life, like the pendulum, leaves infinite transforming spirals in the sands of time. Life is a transformation, not a destination. No one promised that life would be easy or, for that matter, that it would never end.

Love, like paradox, is dualistic. One component exists in a formless, etheric undifferentiated state, while the other takes on form and is more definable and stable. The undefined love, unconditional love, is free from comparison, while the latter, conditional love, is grounded in conditions, judgments and contracts. Yet, both loves share in the common denominator of acceptance and, therefore, in a very significant sense, are not comparable. Unconditional love and conditional love are relative states of a singular love. Neither state exists in absolute purity, for each contains an aspect of the other. Absolute love is like the Taoist mandala of wholeness, which depicts life as a perfect circle created through the duality of opposites. This is represented by the non-colors of black and white, which are equally separated into halves by an "s" wave. Found within the center of each half of the circle is yet another circle that holds its counterpart.

Absolute love is the total sphere which evolves from the interaction of its component parts, while the relative states of its parts (conditional and unconditional) vary with the consciousness of each individual and the society as a whole. Love, as consciousness, evolves towards higher states, but that evolution depends on the tension which is produced through its two aspects. The degree to which we aspire or are absorbed into the unconditional is a result of our personal transcendence of the conditional. Too many conditions or judgments can stifle growth, while an imbalance towards the nonrestrictive, unconditional love or mercy can lead to chaos. Perhaps the highest human attainment is to be poised as if on the "s" wave that separates the paradoxical fields of love, accepting the equalness of both its aspects, and in so doing, unifying it. It is through such balance that we aspire to the singular absolute love. By transforming conditional love into unconditional love, absolute love evolves and so is recycled once again into newer conditions. This is the never-ending life spiral. Creation, like love, is the highest form of alchemy. It is the transmutation of base element into sheer gold.

Eventually, there comes a time in life when we all must transcend duality and assume total responsibility for our own life and fly solo, but the vibration from our wings of decision will be felt throughout the universe and for all eternity. This is a flight that can be taken most harmoniously when we are free from guilt, free from blame, and have acceptance of the past and trust in the present. When self-responsibility is fully accepted, then this moment of truth affords the ideal time to re-enter the process of co-creation—further transformation for ourselves and for those who are to come.

Many couples' difficulties are compounded when two people with different needs attempt to create one form (the child) to fulfill the many requirements in their own lives. Children are too often conceived for societal reasons, as a proof of fertility, as substitute for unfulfilled dreams, as a need to rectify parental injustices, as an attempt for immortality, to preserve a marriage, or to finish a parent's unfinished business. There are an infinite number of conceptions for the wrong reasons. *The immaculate conception is a being that is born free from parental projections.*

If thought indeed dictates form, then how wounding or how constructive is the impact of these intentions, not only to the newborn, but later to the adult? These offspring can live their lives as displaced persons delivered to a hostile planet. The autistic child and the catatonic may represent individuals who have withdrawn from such a hostile environment. Some may say that it is the child's choice. Perhaps it is true that these children have mystically chosen such a barren existence to teach us thoughtfulness. But do we need such severe teachings? Are we that dense, that contracted, that we must be repeatedly reminded, repeatedly reawakened?

If our persistent thought is that our life has not been fulfilled, or that we have not found meaning in our existence, then can we further impose that feeling of deficiency not only on ourselves but on our children and those around us? Now the newborn, throughout life, may try to sort out the disconnected events that preceded its birth. More often than not the child succumbs in bewildered innocence, only to pass that same incompleteness to the next generation.

T. S. Eliot, in *Murder in the Cathedral,* says, "The last temptation is the greatest treason; to do the right deed for the wrong reason."

Is there a right reason for having children? Historically, our forefathers were agrarians and children were conceived not only in love, but as potential laborers to help till and cultivate the soil. Because of the high infant death rate from malnutrition and disease, large families were essential. In those years, children represented personal ownership— possessions the more affluent could not take away. This is still partly true today.

As an intern, I visited an indigent family in New York. I asked the mother of six why she had so many children. Lovingly clutching her youngest, she stated simply, "You can take away my room, my broken TV, my clothes, anything. But you can't take away my children. They're mine." The production of large families has often been sarcastically referred to as "a poor man's entertainment—the poor man's opera." This is understandable as long as the world can give no guarantee to the disadvantaged that the quality of their lives will be changed in any significant way by having fewer children. But the converse of this statement is closer to the truth. As our own quality of *inner* life improves, it is often balanced by a diminished amount of external needs. In either case, who are we to judge another's quality or quantity of love, or even his needs?

If having a child is "a poor man's opera" for some, the drama of a divorce seems to be the rich man's opera for others. This leads to the poignant and urgent question: How do you engender wholeness in a child of an ill-considered marriage or pregnancy? As Rollo May wrote in *The Courage to Create,* ". . . the original trauma which is the source of anxiety is rejection that is lied about." A child is often conceived as bonding glue to strengthen a fractured marriage. The thought, "Perhaps if we have a child . . ." serves as temporary relief for a familial eruption. The couple hopes the child can do for them what they cannot accomplish for themselves. If the child is conceived as the intended savior in this fragile alliance, it is understandable why this same child (at a later date) might feel responsible if this disharmonious relationship continues or fails to continue. Psychologists, psychiatrists, mothers and fathers may attempt to dissuade such children from this inner truth, but, in reality, these children have not fulfilled the preconceptive intention of their parents. The children might not have been the initial cause for the shattered marriage, but it's soon evident that giving birth failed to bond the family together.

True, parents are not entirely responsible for their children's gross interpretations or misinterpretations of life's events. I cannot even deny my own belief that children are involved in the selection of their parents and in the selection of many conditions of their lives. Simply to cast off all the excuses for the negativity of humankind as the grand design of the universe is an escape from responsibility. The responsibility of parents is more than accepting unconditionally the life essence of the newborn that is being expressed through them. Parents, too, can honor the initial contract of their own lives: to be humane. I truly believe if we can maintain the balance of these aspects of love, the conditional and the unconditional, we will have less need for pain as the primary teacher that drives humankind to aspire. Can we resolve our past unfinished business in order to free the energy of conditional love and so tap new levels of a transformational love?

Situations other than a fractured marriage can detract from the initial parental intention of that special moment of lovemaking. One case is of the parent who expects the child to achieve all those things previously denied the parent. The newborn may integrate not only the parents' unfulfilled goals, but also their unfinished societal commitments. The parents' intent to have a child to achieve these ends places an undue stress on the unborn. Even if these goals were set in a loving way, they are, more often than not, misdirected. Could this be a reason why the firstborn is often referred to as the "over-achiever" or (when the pressure becomes too overwhelming for the child) the "dropout"? The comments one hears in the delivery room often reveal how the parents, on occasion, project their desires, fantasies, and frustrations on the newborn:

"Wow! Look at those shoulders! That kid's gonna be one of the great football players of all time!"

". . . with a nose like that, thank God for plastic surgery!"

". . . Whew! Thank Heaven the kid's not bald!"

". . . there she is—Miss America!"

Or what about those people who refer to themselves as "replacement children"? They often were conceived late in their parents' marriage to replace a brother or sister who had died. Their names are usually the same as or similar to that of the sibling who died. The protective restraints placed on these individuals can be oppressive. Often these children become rebellious, or have feelings of guilt—"If my brother had lived, I never would have been here. . . ." Even if they were of a different sex, these children always have the feeling of being compared to that now nonexistent family member. One cannot replace one child with another or, in fact, one object with another. Every aspect of life is unique and yet part of the whole!

I often think of a young woman who died of cancer. The week of her death, a magnificent pine tree, which was situated at the entrance of her home, fell. The pine had filled her family's house with patterns of sunshine and shadow, shade and warmth. After the funeral, they replaced the tree with a huge, fully aged pine. It allows a different quality of sun, a different pattern of shadow into the courtyard. While the tree does not have the same warmth and degree of belonging as the original tree, it still has its own magnificence, its own stateliness, its own life. Evolution does not tolerate sameness. Was the fallen pine a symbol to teach the parents to let go in order to create anew? Was the fallen pine a parable from life itself to teach the family of life's continuum? Was the new pine a symbolic rite of rebirth that helped to salve the pain and cope with the loss?

The quest for immortality is too often expressed through

our children rather than through our own personal living. We are all immortal. Birth and death are only points in time that mark our place, our position, in the universe but which in no way limit the totality of our experiences.

This quest for immortality is sometimes echoed by such a statement as, "Thank God we have a son to carry on the family name of Smith!" The naming of a child can have a profound affect on his or her adult life. The son named after his father might enter a world of comparison, competition, and confusion about his own identity. Little John now waits until Big John is dead before he can become the man his father was or should have been. Too often he lives with guilt for having achieved his dream at his father's death.

Other children are named after a dead relative, a president, or a famous athlete, actor, or actress. Will the '80s show an increase in the number of Dustins, Burts, Farrahs, and Alis, and with these names the implicit assumption of certain talents? The son named "J.P." and offered a choice of becoming a stockbroker, lawyer, or certified public accountant might feel unfulfilled if he preferred to be an artist or a musician or a sailor. The degree to which this might apply would depend, in part, upon the force with which the intention was etched in thought. It might be for this reason that our children have an innate desire to be more than their parents and lose the fact that they innately are.

Perhaps we could learn from "native" cultures, who, rather than projecting, wait and choose a name more in accordance with the child's personality traits, which will become evident after birth. Objectivity is often achieved here by having someone outside the immediate family unit select the name. At a later date, as part of the ceremony of adulthood, the individual can choose his or her name as an act of the co-creative process of transformation. This need for self-expression and identity is illustrated in today's choices of Aquarian-age names like Rainbow, Sunshine, or Flower. These names often reflect the love, hope and unfinished dreams that the parents themselves are searching for as they attempt to integrate more fully with the universe. What does each generation pass to future generations of its intentions, desires, and beliefs, and what do the children bring forth from the yet unknown dimensions of their beingness?

Another reason for having a child might be to fulfill society's implied marriage contract—a contract that only says "to love and honor," but which includes the unspoken "to give birth." Although pregnancy is a biologic fulfillment, it is not necessarily a requirement that must be fulfilled by all couples. The "We've been married for about four years—I guess it's time to have a kid" syndrome does not have to be embraced. In a similar vein, pregnancy can also be launched to float a potential grandparent or to satisfy another type of time requirement. These historical reasons for conceiving are injustices to the creative process.

Other injustices occur when the parents are determined to have a child of a specific sex. To conceive a third child because the prior two were of the same sex is illogical. This inappropriate rationalization, beyond being a major cause of overpopulation, may also be the cause of lifelong confusion as to the child's psychosexual identity. Psychosexual rearing is strongly imprinted by the first eighteen months. If a child of the unwanted sex is born, that child can be driven to strive to fill his or her parents' unspoken wishes.

A woman recently volunteered to me that during World War II she prayed that her child would be a girl because "girls didn't go to war then." Thirty years later her child underwent a transexual operation to become a female. Is this related to parental intention? Is this related to war? Or is this related to the newborn's response to a collective wishful thought of the '40s consciousness? Does thought enhance probability, or is all of life pure coincidence?

I am also reminded of a thirty-year-old, beautifully sensitive woman who was the youngest in a family of three daughters. She told me of her parents' intention and their prayers that this, their third child, would be a boy. She spoke softly, yet emotionally, as she related that as a child her room was decorated with bold, masculine prints, as compared to the feminine room her sisters shared, and how, more often than not, she was dressed in jeans. She gained parental recognition and acceptance through sports and, following high school, she enlisted in the armed forces. Although her present medical complaint is hypertension, her persistent confusion lies in the choices that bisexuality presents. Her depression now rests in the guilt of those choices. To treat her simply with antihypertension medicine would be to afford only incomplete therapy for her chronic self-deprecation, which restricts her every move, thought, and action.

The forms of our children may vary, but their essence is conceived in love—and that is immutable. It is this energy of love that we should strive to channel and then transform into our children and they into us. Is bisexuality a result of misplaced parental intention, or is it unconditional love expressed in physical form? If these same individuals were allowed to emit their innermost feelings, free from societal judgments, would this love be more likely to exist in its formless unconditional state than in its physical state? Is the prebirth form of our existence in a stage of unconditional love? Is this love transformed in the fires of conditional life? In love's attempt to be reborn, does it so evolve to greater heights through the life experience? I think so, but again, is it necessary for the judgment of society to be so abrasive if that love is manifested physically? I think not.

The case histories, as presented throughout this book, are not told to promote parental guilt but parental understanding. Not only these individuals, but all of us and all of humanity, are active participants in our own creation. Our choices are not to be judged as to right or wrong, good or bad, or to be blamed on others. If we understand the influences in our lives, then perhaps we can accept our choices and our results with less anxiety and pain. In the final analysis, we are still the ones who choose to act out our parental thoughts and societal judgments. It, therefore, behooves both parents and society to present clearer options and fewer judgments. It is time for society to recognize that the hopes and dreams of parents need not be spoken. Thoughts are transmitted at the speed of light and with the intensity of a penetrating laser.

A woman wrote me the following paragraph after reading one of my papers on pregnancy and unconditional love:

"I confess that my own initial reaction in the beginning of your paper, beneath the genuine interest in content—was a constant low-grade anxiety. What do you mean, unconditional love? Does 'complete acceptance of all life's interactions and transactions' include moments when I hate my child, my initial ambivalence about his conception, my very unmotherly feelings of wanting to bash his head against the radiator when he gets me up six times in one night? Is that 'love'? It doesn't seem like love; indeed, I like myself least when I snap at David or lose my temper with him, even though I know I'm human, that I do genuinely adore him most of the time, and that small children can be exasperating. Are all people capable of unconditional love? Or is it only a goal to strive for but one never to be truly reached?"

I don't know anyone who is in a constant pure state of unconditional love. As I stated earlier, the unconditional holds within it the conditional. However, humankind is on the threshold of comprehending the transforming power of thought. Soon we will realize that, with the acceptance of our humanness which was founded in love, there will be less need for forgiveness, apologies, or guilt. This does not negate our responsibility for our actions. It means that we will have become more aware of ourselves, of our thoughts, and so more responsive to others. Acceptance of our humanness is the first step on the path to embracing unconditional love. Unconditional love is not reserved just for others, it begins with one's self.

Humankind will soon appreciate that the pure intention of love followed by the action of love are the seeds for creative interchange. The will to hold fast the power of this intention until the creation—our child—is delivered into a similar perfection is the never-ending task of all humankind.

I am reminded of Richard Bach's statement in his book *Illusions:* "Here is a test to find whether your mission on earth is finished. If you are alive, it isn't."

Thought can shape form. But if it is true, as the Taoists say, that "the only constant in life is change," then you have the power to create change at any moment of your life. It is precisely that movement toward change that initiates transformation for you and your child. If our initial intent or action was, indeed, poorly conceived, then the present moment provides adequate time to rectify it. Thought is not set immutably in stone. It is only non-thought that leads to stagnation and constancy.

At the same time, negative events or thoughts cannot and should not always be avoided. The powerful energy generated from the friction of this learning experience decreases the likelihood for that test to be repeated again. The neuroanatomist knows well that the appreciation and recall of pain is essential for survival; these experiences have evolved multiple access routes to the brain to insure its long-term memory, and with that recall, the appropriate response for avoidance learning. You don't have to tell a child twice not to touch the hot stove. So, too, negative events can indelibly imprint memory and thereby serve as effective positive teachers of life.

Pain can be considered the sixth sense. Pain's sharp, cutting quality which is characteristic of blocked energy makes it palpable and definitely memorable, while love is so subtle and fluid that its evanescent quality barely imprints short-term memory. Humankind's quest is to convert the pathways of the brain's emotional recall from the sixth sense of pain to that of love.

Love is a great teacher, but since it tends to be ephemeral, it demands our focused attention over time. Once we learn how to sustain love, we will have less need to learn from acute bouts of pain. However, often in the unmasking of our discomfort we are pleasantly shocked to find that the love was disguised as pain just to get our undivided attention. I believe that the opposite of love is pain; each, again, contains an element of the other.

Can we differentiate between what can and cannot be changed, and then accept the wisdom of our choice and, yes, the wisdom that comes through the uneasiness of our helplessness? Can we learn compassion for ourselves and others and recognize: each individual and event (even if painful) is but our teacher—and we, in turn, are also the teachers of others and those who are to follow? It is hoped the "parent-to-be" can reflect for a time on the mental, physical, and spiritual conditions which surrounded his or her own birth. The wisdom gained from such insight may provide a clearer definition of self. This is the first step for birth without fear.

It is never too late to reflect on the past in order to accept the present and to prepare more fully for the future. The desire to honor life with life and to transform love into form is the reason to create—the reason for children—our *Gift to Life.*

Pregnancy now becomes not only the metaphor for transformation, but is a master teacher for the learning of the perfection in all things. The purer our focused thought, the more translucent will be the thread of love that runs through all humanity. Thoughts, too, labor!

A student of mine wrote the following poem:

A Gift of Love

Alone
is nice.
Loneliness
isn't
(except when we recognize it as fertile soil
for growth which we recognize later and
meanwhile)

Loneliness is
painful.
Even the recollection of lonely, isolated,
touch-less times hurts.

I do not know if
two months of isolation
at birth
without bonding
causes me to feel separated and different
from my family

Has the child in me been cared for so I can
grow
into an adult?

I do know
I need to be held
(husband holding doesn't count and
I don't know why)

I do know
if you want my attention,
touch me
I do know
when I am in the grip of
loneliness, anguishing inside and still persevering
I don't know
(does anyone? Everyone?)
how to get what I need
to move on.

If I could
give myself me
I would be giving
a gift of love.

Melanie '78

The entire process of self-acceptance can be carried out prior to conception. We cannot share in the birth of a perfect child until we first give birth to the perfection that has existed silently but patiently in our own lives. The shared creation, you and your child, are gifts of love to and from the universe—gifts that can be free of parental needs, expectations, projections, and conditions. But we cannot give birth to such an immaculate conception until we first give birth to that understanding within ourselves.

In the end, life is a contract and so imposes the required responsibilities not only on the couple but on all humankind. Each being is called forth to share in the unfolding of life's "ultimate investment." The words of Laura Huxley ring loud and clear: "Our children are indeed our ultimate investment." But if this is true, then so are the parents. We are all children and parents interacting with one another. Each soul is born in thought and then is transformed through the contract and contact of life.

Pregnancy is humankind's greatest gift to humanity; yet it is its greatest risk. To conceive or not to conceive is indeed the primary question. It precedes "to be" or "not to be." The thought to conceive or not to conceive is invariably fraught with tension; however, the tension created in that choice has the power to affect not only your child, but yourself and, in fact, all humankind. If we could stop for but only a moment to reflect upon the power of each of our thoughts, and the transformation of these thoughts to form, it would be too overwhelming and, yes, too frightening for most of us to withstand.

The power of our formless, yet focused, thought can penetrate the resistant, yet total, potential void of our unconsciousness prior to our decision to conceive or not to conceive. In its literal sense, it is as if thought were struck by hand, manifested, in order to reveal itself more clearly to the creator and to those who share in the creation. Thought is the beginning that has no end. Thought gives birth to the eternal thread of life that supports the transformational process called a shared creation. Thought is *The Word.*

It is never too late to offer affirmations to those who still live or those who have died, to all eternal beings who still await to be more clearly defined by our love.

Pregnancy is the metaphor that gives form to that word— *Love.*

III | One must first begin with oneself.

In The Beginning

Past • Present • Future
Holographic/Biocomputer Mind

The act of conception can be compared with two pebbles that are simultaneously thrown into a clear placid lake. The moment each pebble touches the water's surface is equivalent to the birth of the husband's and the wife's thoughts to conceive. Now, as the farthest wave from the center of one stone's impact reaches the corresponding ripple of the other, there is a coming, a merging, and a fusing into one. The form of the new wave, the child, depends, in part, on the individual frequencies of each parent's thought and each parent's genetic code at the moment of union.

Therefore, it is from the multiple points of interaction between the formless thoughts and the formed genetic codes that the hologram of birth takes place. From these interacting disparate waves the newborn energy is transmuted into form, while the form of husband and wife is transformed into parenthood. Creation is the result of the transaction that arises from interacting participants. As a result of this union, change has irrevocably occurred and the couple and the child have been permanently altered by the act of creation, as has been the surface upon which they have been cast—life.

The phenomena of interaction, union, and creation are found through the natural and the physical sciences. As subatomic particles collide, they are annihilated; yet at the very moment of death, they give birth to a new set of particles.

The willingness to accept the outcome of creative risk and its byproduct, change, be it birth or the change from wife to mother or husband to father, as a result of the act of conception, is a personal choice. However, although marriage and pregnancy are contracts designed by choice, the universe will never ever be the same as a result of that choice. The contract of life is irrevocably eternal and unaltered by death, divorce, or separation.

Physics again offers us a metaphor for the working through of life's contracts. Light, like love, has dualistic properties. Light is both a wave and a particle. The particle is identified by fixing the basic unit of light, a photon, to either its past or its future position. The wave, on the other hand, speaks to the photon's uninterrupted momentum between events and so represents the evolving now.

If this can be seen in relation to our own lives, then the more our position in life is fixed by the conditions of our past or where we expect to be in the future, the less distance we travel in the evolving wave of now.

The inescapable events of conception, birth, and death are absolute contracts in time that are shared by all humankind. These momentous, fixed events, in a sense, mark and define our position and existence in the dimension of chronologic time, while the frequency of the waves that separate these historic events is human time. All life labors. Our own personal labor pattern is a wave of peaks and valleys produced by life's mini-conditions and contracts and their respective resolutions and acceptance. The continuum of this spiral wave is the thread of the life process. Each wave adds to the evolving shared creation called life. The more we accept unconditionally the conditions of our lives, the more quality we experience in our own lives and the more distance we personally travel in humantime and the evolving now. The acceptance of life's pain of labor gives birth to life's love for life.

If it is true that the child is father to the man, then we

need to ask what were the conditions in our own lives. What was my labor? Who were the role models who shaped my existence? What were my parents' choices in life? Where was their nourishment? Can it be that some of the parental beatings—verbal or even physical—have been meted out by those who desperately wanted their infants to become more than they were? "God, I hope my children don't turn out like me!" Or, "I want you to be more than I am, damn it!" This self-destructive chastisement is so often inappropriately expressed in words and deeds.

The parents of battered babies are not mutant strains but, more often than not, they too suffered through and were tempered by a hostile environment. Now, years later, as parents, they are acting out what to them was once a familiar pattern. On the other hand, some may argue that one way to learn love is to be placed in an environment where acceptance is difficult to find. There must be a better way. The fire of life itself will provide enough fuel for growth.

As the parents' and child's life energies of force and resistance fuse, this union provides the relative friction that is needed to transform what once was to what is: the newborn, the new woman, and the new man. However, if our combined energies are too highly charged or too weak, then this imbalance can be abortive for the parents as well as the child, or at least too repressive for growth. It is as if the scale has tipped too far to one pole and remains fixed. As the parents share in the creation of the child, the child, too, shares in the movement of the parent toward adulthood.

Many of life's injustices that are experienced by parents and children during periods of maximum stress are easier to view less judgmentally after they have passed. At a later date, these same stresses may be judged to be an essential step in growth and development. In the future, perhaps we will learn to be less judgmental of the present as we appreciate the orderliness and purpose of the past. Perhaps the child of the future will be born out of a balance of both unconditional and conditional love and thus into a world of total acceptance. This would mark a quantum change in human consciousness.

Now may be the time to reflect and question: If I am a co-creator in my own existence, why did I ever choose *those* parents? What am I to learn from *this* life's existence, and is this experience dependent on those parents?

Perhaps your mother and father were inept, total nonentities, or even better, the most obnoxious individuals on earth, just to provide the needed milieu, the fertilizer, for your personal growth. Are they the Buddha in disguise or are you the Buddha for their learning experience?

Evolution depends on the interaction of subtle differences but what appears to be pure coincidence or chance always evolves towards order. Coincidence is the temporary teacher, the elementary school teacher who prepares us for graduate work. What responses were made to the coincidences within your life? What have you gained through those quirk happenstances? In such a context, coincidence exists in relative time; however, in absolute time (the continuum of all time), it assumes its rightful, orderly place.

Adulthood is not a gift of age but is a stage in life when an individual unconditionally accepts the coincidences of life as being perfect.

The Egyptians had a wonderful phrase to express the order, commonality, and interconnectedness in all things: "As above, so below." If we could literally apply this to ourselves, we would find that everything in life obeys the same laws of order. Perhaps we could for a moment imagine ourselves as subatomic particles swimming in a physicist's bubble chamber. If now the physicist were to photograph us within the chamber, capture us in relative time, we would be identified in the massive sea of particles by the unique configuration of the path of our past—doctor, lawyer, or carpenter.

Dr. Sid Drell, director of Stanford Linear-Accelerator Center, would say, "The idea is to find the pattern and the game is simple." In a real sense, we are mere particles defined by the stimuli and responses of our past, playing in the evolving game of life. So, too, the observed particle is a reflection of the rebirth that occurs from the innumerable stresses and deaths of its past. We are no different from those particles. Einstein wrote in his thesis on *Relativity,* "All phenomena of nature, all the laws of nature, are identical for all systems moving uniformly, relative to each other." And in an earlier paper on *Brownian Movement,* which dealt with the random movement of suspended particles, Einstein described the following:

"Examination of a particle, say, every thirty seconds, reveals the fantastic form of its path. The amazing thing is the apparently eternal character of the motion." He explained this phenomenon as being due to the kinetic energy (motion) of the invisible molecules with which they were constantly colliding. In a sense, was Einstein, in determining the cause of the particles' agitation, acting as the particles' psychiatrist?

In physics, these unseen particles are identified by certain properties and behaviors: "spin," "change," "charm," and "strangeness," and in the future, perhaps "truth" and "beauty." Molecular physics, the study of "the unseeable," is reminiscent of Hebrews 11:3: "By faith we understand that the universe was created at God's command, so that what we now see was made out of what cannot be seen." We can readily give names to unseen particles and accept their presence but have incredible difficulty with the likes of God and Love. The total trust in science yet the lack of trust in faith (acceptance without the need to understand) is to me indeed "strangeness."

In either case, if we can now imagine ourselves rising above the physicist's bubble chamber and review our past from afar, there is the possibility that the path that identifies us can be brought into clearer view—under conscious control.

What are the stimuli and the responses of your past that have brought you to question whether to conceive or not to conceive or even to be born? After intensive soul searching, you may be better prepared to answer these questions and, in so doing, you can become an active orchestrator of your existence, rather than a helpless particle in space who blames the outer world for its lot in life.

If it is true that with every force there is an equal and opposite force, then you can begin to control the responses to the forces of your life and consciously effect a probability of change. The understanding of the universe that comes through the working through of our unique trials, tribulations, and insights are the gifts we bequeath to all the children of the universe. These gifts are our immortality.

Before conception is the ideal time for this self-reflection, the time to explore the various interactions of your brain, an intellect which, until now, has shielded and protected you from self-discovery.

The science of laser photography, holography, provides us with a scientific model to study both creation and the creative mind. To produce this three-dimensional photographic image (known as a hologram), a laser, coherent light source, is split into two beams—a working beam and a reference beam. The working beam is directed to the object to be photographed and then is deflected to a developing plate where it interfaces (merges) with its co-creator, the second beam. The second beam, or reference beam, reaches the same plate directly, without being obstructed by any object. The holographic plate, therefore, is a composite of interface patterns created from a single source of light.

At the same time, each fragment of the formed plate holds within it the entire memory of the hologram. When a laser is passed through either the whole photographic plate, or even one of its fragments, the image photographed is reproduced in space as an illusion of the initial subject. The light that is needed to produce the holographic plate, and later to reproduce the image, the laser, is reminiscent of the story of creation—*Genesis.*

"Let there be light!" Light is split; one segment maintains the uninterrupted quality of the source, love, while the other meets the resistant earth. At the point of impact between the force (light) and resistance (earth), a new form emerges when radiated by its source (love), and rising from the settling dust, we see that form to be human. In the Bible, creation takes place in the transformation of the formless into the form, while laser photography transforms form into the formless. Both, however, share in the same source of transformation—Light.

The etheric source of formless love and the grounding strength and stability of Mother Earth speak to the origin and integration of the formless and formed aspects of humankind which unite to become the essential spirit that flows through us, our children, and all creations of the universe.

Humankind's illusion is based on viewing itself solely in form—in the apparent, in the observable—that reflects light, rather than in its other aspect, the formless—the transparent—whose diaphanous state allows light through. This is also a source of creation. Creation is born from the integration of both the form and the formless.

Physics is no different from religion, nor is biology distinct from philosophy or art. So, too, the sperm and the ovum share in common ground but are defined or conditioned into their unique aspects. All aspects of life are no more than a hologram converging upon a hologram: force within resistance; sperm within egg, parent within child, and conditional love within unconditional love. The entire holographic process is life itself. However, in the transformational process, the converging holograms produce a new form, a new hologram, and thereby the quality of humankind evolves within a singular source of All energy.

As any singular isolated human cell has the potential to clone the entire organism, so, too, to understand one thing is to see its reflection in all things. Just as one fragment of the holographic plate has the memory of the entire picture within it, every aspect of life has found within it the story of all life.

The human mind houses a holographic image of reality that reflects both our personal world and the universal world. Sigmund Freud proposed that the re-evoking of a memory trace of a perception becomes equivalent to the re-establishment of the situation of original satisfaction or dissatisfaction and, thereby, the wish is fulfilled. In describing hysteria, Freud notes, "It not infrequently happens that, instead of a singular major trauma, we found a number of partial traumas forming a group of provoking causes."

Our life's illusions of people and events are housed together within our minds. Each thought and act is entwined and eternally stored in our memory, waiting to be either reflected, projected, or retrieved by key circumstances of the present. Even illusionary perceptions can trigger exaggerated chains of emotional and physical reactions.

The units that comprise the brain, neurons, fortunately have the unique quality of plasticity. Therefore, memory circuits can be altered by either the addition or the re-evaluation of new thoughts and events in our lives. Relearning takes place through the constant repetition of these new thoughts and actions of our lives over a period of time. This does not entirely erase memory but offers us new choices to the stimuli of our lives. We really have the power to reprogram our mind's perceptions, and thus, our responses.

However, since any experience which is perceived can leave behind a memory trace which has a potential of becoming associated with other experiences, then the recall of any part of an experience can rekindle the entire memory process, or engram. This is identical to the holographic model. Time also can alter the apparent clarity of events and effect misunderstanding. Events of humankind are not static or linear but obey the law of a space-time continuum. Humankind's self-imposed expectations plus the weight of other people and conditions within our life can warp our understanding of reality. The dimension of chronologic time allows the interval between cause and effect to be filled with noncausal events such as rewards, punishments, and coincidences. In such an interaction, noncausality effects causality and our view of reality.

If it is true that we are the composite of all previous experiences, then this could explain why many patients report prenatal and delivery experiences similar to those of their mothers. Dr. David Cheek, an obstetrician, uses hypnosis as a method to unlock hidden fears of pregnancy and often helps his patients uncover stories about their own traumatic births. He has noticed that during regression hypnosis, adults perform head and shoulder movements identical to those displayed by the unborn during birth as it unfolds like a flower from a state of perfect flexion to extension—lifting its head gently at the end of the birth process to be received and welcomed.

These observations are similar to those of Stanislav Grof. He tells us that during LSD psychotherapy, cancer patients re-experience movements identical to the birthing process. Both authors feel these early moments of life are permanently imprinted and stored in the long-term memory banks of our minds. Their conclusions are consistent with accounts from individuals who claim to have re-experienced their delivery in isolation tanks or during "rebirthing" exercises as described by Leonard Orr and Sondra Ray. Doctor Arthur Janov even describes the reappearance of traumatic marks on the face of an adult patient who was re-experiencing birth during primal therapy.

A case comes to mind of a young woman in her twenties who, for the past five years, has been living with her cancer. Since childhood, she has experienced a choking feeling when she becomes emotionally overwhelmed. When I asked her about the circumstances of her birth, she casually stated, "Oh, I was born with a cord around my neck—damn near died." Could that earliest event of life now be associated with the size and consistency of the malignant lymph nodes around her neck, nodes which seem to fluctuate in size as much with her psychological state as they do with her chemotherapy? In either case, she now uses these same "lumps" that once produced fear and panic as a weather vane of both her physical and mental environment that seeks detente. Her cancer has become her internal psychiatist.

I recently saw a frail, thirty-year-old woman who suffered with anorexia nervosa. This is a condition in which a person eats barely enough food for maintenance while at other times he or she obsessively gorges on food after which they induce vomiting. Such a being soon begins to take on the appearance of a famine victim because of this self-denial. When I first met my patient, she was painfully thin, drawn, and depressed. Dryly, without emotion, she related that she was the second of two children and blandly told how she was born to a mother who openly expressed unhappiness about conceiving her so soon after the birth of her first child. Her mother told her how she prayed that she would either abort the pregnancy or have a stillborn.

Could it be that that mother's intention is now being fulfilled thirty years later as her daughter slowly wastes away through self-imposed deprivation of food and love? My client now thrives on rejection, which has become so familiar to her that she actually seeks out interpersonal relationships that are nonnourishing or are so volatile as to be short lived. These relationships validate her earliest life impressions that the universe is hostile, nonsupporting, and noncaring. Her overeating is an attempt to gain nourishment, while her forced vomiting is her declaration that "I am unworthy to survive," a statement acted upon through repeated suicide attempts and a resistance to enter a long-term relationship or to have children of her own.

In truth, her mother's desire not to carry the pregnancy may have stemmed from, not lack of love, but love. Her mother feared her own ability to be a nourishing mother. Her mother, who is now in her late fifties, also seeks nourishment—the same nourishment that was denied to her during her own childhood. She, too, had no role model, no template for parenthood.

Our past is often the template that is transmitted from generation to generation to insure that eventually one family member gets the message to change. When that individual lives the resolution to that specific problem, the entire universe resounds in joy. All who have preceded are part of the lesson to be learned and thereby partake in its resolution. We all benefit, for we are all interrelated.

Implicit in every parent-child relationship is love but, unfortunately, it is all too often hidden from view and distorted through time. My thirty-year-old friend, in reviewing both her mother's and her own past, and by acknowledging her own role in maintaining her self-destructive path, is gradually overcoming both the external and internal malnourishment in her life. Can it be that her mother was the necessary pawn for this insight? Is it possible that as this young woman taps her unlimited love that she will also be nourishing not only herself, but healing her mother and all of humanity? I think so.

In these two case histories, we can see how confusing signals may enter the receptive holographic mind of not only the newborn but the yet unborn and be carried into the thoughts and actions of that child's adulthood. It is also within the holographic model that we understand how the interrelationships of causal and noncausal events can fuse as if to complete a specific design. This is what Carl Jung refers to as synchronicity.

The intensity of the emotion evoked from the recall of any fragment of the past is often heightened by the number of previous similar memories that the emotion triggers. Perhaps the increase in the intensity of emotion occurs in order to make the message so blatant that its meaning cannot be ignored.

Dr. Viktor E. Frankl, noted psychiatrist and author, wrote: "If a person has found a meaning to his life, that person will accept whatever fate he meets. The person will accept suffering, give sacrifice and even his life. But if there is no meaning in his existence, that person is just as likely to take his own life, even when surrounded by plenty." What is your path? What is your meaning?

The more parents and children communicate about the events that enveloped the circumstances of birth and those early years (both for parents and child), the greater the hope is of healing wounds. The key to healing is through a mutually understandable form of communication. If we can talk, we can perhaps touch emotionally, perhaps make contact with our past, with ourselves, and with each other. This type of dialogue has the power to unravel the disparity in beliefs that can separate people, a separation that is brought about through the inconsistencies of language and the warp of time. Time can be equated with distance, and so, too, in life we find that a prolonged breakdown in understanding can cause a distancing between people which often obscures their "meaning to life."

Paul Courderc's statement, "The interval between two events presents a more profound reality than the events themselves," was written about atomic physics. But time and space now take on a significant meaning in the explanation of our most common misunderstandings of love. Love is too often only experienced in the moments when we touch, but love can be felt without touching and spoken in silence. Unfortunately, the warp produced in the space-time continuum of life is more often than not filled with our expectations and our misinterpretations. Our future is usually the unfinished business of our past.

The events of history can also affect our decisions and intentions concerning birth and life. They are also lessons that are too often forgotten and so must be replayed. Since humankind resists change, these events, too, keep increasing in severity. The holocaust that took place only forty years ago is a document to how reticent humankind is to learn and then to change. Since that epoch in history, "man's inhumanity to man" has hardly diminished. The truth of this statement can be found on the front page of today's newspaper.

Was it all in vain? What is our personal threshold or our collective maximum tolerance to the pain of war before we get the message and surrender in love? Dr. Frankl, who survived the holocaust of the concentration camps, has also written: "Remember, it was mankind that designed and built the ovens and the gas chambers of the concentration camps, and it was also mankind that walked into those ovens with human dignity and a prayer on the lips."

Perhaps those prayers were, in part, unanswered and did not go unnoticed. The Viet Nam war flower children were but pregnant thoughts in the '40s. The post-World War II baby boom was partly prompted by a realization of humankind's mortality and was an attempt at immortality. It is understandable why the progeny would seek to fulfill the pregnant parental intention, "I hope my child doesn't go to war," by joining in anti-war demonstrations, ecology causes, and the like.

The gap that exists between these two generations may be more the result of parental intention now dulled and diminished through passage of time and affluence than any real ideological differences. Is it possible the parents' previous peace-seeking thoughts may have impregnated their fetuses before birth? Was this generation driven relentlessly beyond their own control to carry placards to stop the war? This is also the generation that has come to realize less might be more—a generation that defers marriage and childbearing to later years, a generation of veterans whose psychological scars of war are still undergoing debridement.

The students during the Korean conflict were preteens during World War II and viewed the war in Europe and the Pacific through the eyes and ears of Hollywood movies. To them, the Korean war was not judged as to its morality, but as a potential impediment to their education. These students were conceived in the early Roosevelt years and they shared in adulthood some of the same fears as did their depression-conscious parents—financial insecurity. While members of this generation do not rock the boat, they also prefer not to scratch the Mercedes. Our history is carried into the present and future. Events of the past can produce stress-filled situations whose origins are buried in time. Apparently unrelated events can become almost insurmountable hurdles for the unborn, for the newborn, or for the adult. These events are coming at such a rapid frequency that generations are being demarcated by decades or less rather than by scores. Eventually we will no longer be able to forget or escape our past inhumanity.

My sister and brother-in-law, who were married in 1943, provide a good example. By the time my sister delivered her first child in 1944, Elliot, her husband, was in the Pacific. Upon his return to the states, he was reluctant to talk about his experiences. When I hounded him as any twelve-year-old can do, he finally screamed, "There is no such thing as a good war!"

His son, Andy, graduated from college twenty years later during the Viet Nam war. Andy represented the Aquarian. He was exquisitely sensitive to the needs of his fellow man and communed with Mother Earth through poetry and other writings. I can still see him, on his sixteenth birthday, lying in a canoe reading Whitman's *Leaves of Grass.* He was noticeably anguished four years later by the incomprehensibility of war. Andy was essentially given no choice. He could choose between being a soldier or an escapee to Canada.

To assuage his confusion and in an attempt to find temporary asylum, Andy went to Mexico. A month later, I, too, went to the Mexican town of Puerto Vallarta, but it was to claim Andy's drowned body—a body wracked more by the thoughtless choice of others than by the effects of water intoxication. Andy was conceived during a mother's fears that her husband might never see their child, and born into a father's vibration which carried the mental scars of even "the most just and moral of all wars." By the time of Andy's birth, the newborn babe was already a war victim. Are we ready to welcome the eternal energy of Andy's innocence and love back into the '80s?

The thoughts and prayers of the '40s were received but still remain only partially answered. This book is written to make not only the reader but myself more cognizant of how short our memories are of "never again" and how imperative it is to honor our initial intentions of pregnancy—to give life to life, not to diminish it.

Even today, there are holocausts within what Buckminster Fuller fondly calls "Spaceship Earth," but one can hope that now we will begin to evolve toward that greater meaning to life. I cannot help but feel that the energy of today's parental thoughts have merged with the eternal energy of those who died with "human dignity" in all the holocausts of war and in so doing have given birth to "The Age of Aquarius." Those souls, in the fiery deaths of war, willed us a new quality of life. Can we accept their gift? Can we welcome their children? Can we begin today?

Whether the teacher is one of joy or sorrow, pain or pleasure, our responses and rebirths must be recognized as having been triggered as much by the hologram of our individual and collective past as by the present. The questions then become: Can old signals be heeded sooner, modified, or even prevented entirely? Is there a less painful teacher than war? Can we become aware of our own intention to be born and honor those conditions and contracts? If so, we can begin to follow those most orderly signposts that guide us and those which lead toward a more harmonious present.

When I listen to patients as they present their autobiographies, I have a feeling that many of life's events are conjured up to provide each of us with another chance to work through our unique tasks and intents in life. If a new chance is missed, then often the next lesson becomes more painful than the one before. Each time, the lessons become less escapable until the code of our past is deciphered in the harmony of the present experience. Resolution is that point of understanding which is achieved in life when it is no longer necessary for us to repeat the past, but to only experience the unfolding present.

In such a context, the past is perfect, as it is the repository of the lessons to be learned, while the present offers us fresh choices which will be affected by how well we have done our homework. If the past continues to be unresolved, then the future is no more than a replay of our incomplete past experience. The discrepancy between where one is in the present and where one wishes to be in either the past or the future is the degree to which one suffers.

Ideally, with acceptance, the past will hold less power. Then, each moment in the present will offer a new creative experience—a new beginning, free from unfinished business. As the past fades, the present finally becomes perfect. There is no longer even a future but only *the evolving now*. Even though some may argue that life is a gamble and that even the chick must peck through the resistant shell in order to survive, I believe that a child conceived in a state that is free from parental expectations will be more attuned to the life experience. This child will be less likely to begin a life that is shrouded in the loose threads of its parents' unfinished vestments. Parenthood begins prenatally by gaining insights into oneself, thereby completing the various stages of life that lead inevitably to adulthood and, if chosen, parenthood.

And so, the past is honored in its completion and now the past can serve as a stable foundation for a new creation and a personal transformation.

The unforeseeable personal traumas of life will produce enough fertilizer for growth. A case in point that relates to those impressionable first months of life is that of a strong, vibrant, down-to-earth woman in her mid-thirties who consulted me because of painful joints dating back twelve years to the time of her divorce. She had been hospitalized only once before in her life and that was for meningitis when she was ten months old. It was interesting to me that her present joint pain was aggravated when I moved her neck and legs through those same motions that I would have used to test for meningitis. Was it possible that her divorce recalled an old memory pattern of the isolation or abandonment imposed by her childhood infectious meningitis? Was this specific emotion, the fear of isolation, intimately connected with a thirty-year-old memory of pain-wracked extremities? Could this be the real cause of her present arthritic condition, or could this also be a mechanism for secondary gain, affection?

My friend related how hard she worked throughout her childhood to overcome her limp and its physical limitations caused by the meningitis. She spoke of how she had been praised for overcoming this handicap and how eagerly she sought and cherished parental approval for her accomplishments. Perhaps this explains her choice of a career—that of a physical education teacher. Perhaps the need for the warmth of this repeated kind of praise was what drove her relentlessly to teach sports despite her exquisite pain. Was this why she sought out activities like jogging, skiing, and volleyball, which would aggravate her present condition? Is this why she prides herself on being a teacher who has an innate ability to develop "strength" and "character" in her students?

Although the events of severe isolation and the rewards that went with it were separated by thirty years, she has gained understanding of the relationship between this time/space sequence and has been able to gain insight into her emotional and physical pain. Now, for the first time, she understands (and, more importantly, accepts) her parents, her husband, and friends more fully. She has made significant changes in her personal life. She has begun to use the pain in her joints as a reminder of her destructive drive to achieve and as an indication to respond to life's stimuli in a more transformational manner than through illness. She now uses her pain to remind herself to stop, reflect, and to readjust creatively her "now" to a more pleasurable state, one based on self-approval and love. Her pain has become her internal psychiatrist. She has balanced her need to motivate her students to accomplish with an equal acceptance of both their and her own limitations. She demonstrates well how fragments of the past, when understood and acted upon, can provide the seeds for rebirth and change. Reincarnation is in the here and now.

Although many such stories can only be considered as anecdotal (that is, recountable as an experience but not scientifically proven), we should still be aware that there is a possibility that every incident is indelibly imprinted upon our minds. Physicians, parents, and society, in general, can begin to acknowledge how important the seemingly insignificant noncausal events that surround birth can program an individual at the earliest age and how these same events share a lifetime of their own within that person. Each life story is a significant teaching for all humankind and cannot be evaluated in terms of statistics alone. As E. E. Cummings said,

"I'd rather learn from one bird how to sing
Than teach ten thousand stars how not to dance."

But changes do not always unfold blithely and easily just because of the enlightenment following such reflective processes. People may have profound insight related to their present behavior and still remain stuck in despair. Movement is more often subtle and so life simmers slowly in order to insure a more lasting flavor through experiencing feelings and emotions of both the past and the present and through being allowed to express these in a nonthreatening environment. At times, we may even need the assistance of a therapist to act as a muted mirror image for this sorting-out process. At other times, to solve our personal paradox is often to live it. Whatever path in life we select can serve as a teacher, a teacher that may be judged only as to the relative joy or relative suffering we experience, but should never be compared to the importance of the lesson learned.

Referring once again to my own autobiography: if I can assume that one of my many tasks in life is to learn the balance between hopefulness and helplessness, what could be a more appropriate stimulus to be a physician than the death of my best friend at age ten? I fantasized that if I had been with my friend, Buddy, I would have saved him from his death. The next twenty-three years of my life were devoted to two purposes—saving lives and battling death.

What parents could be more fitting for my life's dream than a father whose earliest ambitions were to be a physician but who, due to his life circumstances, was limited to a sixth-grade education, a father who would sacrifice anything to see his son as a doctor? I was delivered to a mother whose first child, a male, died at birth, and into a family of two sisters who offered me constant love and affection. Was this my impetus to be an obstetrician-gynecologist?

I am reminded of my mother's hopefulness: "Paul, you can accomplish anything you want in life." But I also remember the source of my helplessness when I stood by my father's bedside following his cancer surgery. I watched him die as the nurses called in vain for medical assistance, yet refused me the appropriate medicine to administer to him. I was just six months away from receiving my medical degree. Was this why I took specialty training in cancer surgery? This is but one of the many lessons within my own life that taught me to live with my helplessness. If I did not learn from my experience with my friend and my father, then I had other chances to learn more about the paradox of hopefulness and helplessness as that cancer surgeon.

I am still in the process of learning those things I can change and accepting those that I cannot. I am learning that I am impotent to save or destroy anything. I am reminded of being awakened in the middle of the night, just a few years ago, by a voice that firmly said: "The only one who can save you is you." However, although I may be at times helpless to change the quantum of another's life, I now unquestioningly believe that my life as well as yours does effect the quality of all existence.

That may be why after a forty-four year odyssey I left the formal practice of obstetrics and gynecology to counsel people with cancer and at the same time write a book on birth. *Life is A Shared Creation* is my attempt to resolve my chosen paradox: hopefulness in the face of helplessness. All our lives are worth sharing and in one way or another, each one of us is asked to write our own bible and to risk in the sharing of our Life's understanding.

Who is competent enough to judge or even save another? Who are the sick and who are the well? What is the quality of that human's life? There are figuratively millions of people who have been subjected to the ravages of inhumanity or the unpredictable natural occurrences of life. Yet these survivors often possess a zest for and an understanding of life that transcends knowing. Do they create their own reality? Is their reality as valid as ours? Is life but a personal myth and is reality but society's consensus of a given myth?

If our reality is, in part, an illusion, then why not create an experience of the universe that works for you? In the final analysis, the only one who can transform you is you, and perhaps the only thing you can ever change in life is your perception of yourself. Others may affect you but only if you accept their offering.

In chemistry, we know that a basic element cannot be altered by changing the number of electrons which surround it. When this occurs, it is referred to as an isotope of the basic element. However, when the proton mass of an element, the inner matrix, is altered, then and only then does the true nature of the element change, as does the electron universe that surrounds it. This metaphor is found throughout life. Even the surgeon knows that a wound heals from inside out—one must begin with oneself, we cannot ask the world to change first.

We are exquisite beings who can heal ourselves and our universe by first changing ourselves and so transmuting our original form to yet another. Yet in that incredible act of letting go of the familiar, the universe will forever be transformed by our singular act of change. The power of individual transformation is awesome. Transformation that is free from comparisons and judgments is preparation for giving birth to form, to ourselves and our child. Change is not easy. Even in particle physics, as the physicist tries to alter a singular particle within an aggregate of particles, the force to hold together "what was" gets stronger. Change, transformation, is our challenge, our work, our reason for being. This takes the courage to be you.

The potential for rebirth, or "the coming home," in what is more commonly referred to as "this lifetime," is infinite. To wait for the mystical "next time around" may be to miss the golden ring on the carousel. Perhaps you can ask yourself a few questions. Who am I? Why was I born? Am I living a paradox? What is my personal myth and how did I create it? How did my choice of parents meet these needs? How did I meet theirs? How did the events of my life further or decrease the probability that I would learn these lessons? What beliefs am I to transcend, if, at all, any? Why am I here to receive and what am I here to give?

I have a very wise, 86-year-old friend who challenges me incessantly: "To question is a privilege—to answer is the privilege of the question." Life offers you the questions. You are the answers. The answers to the many questions concerning yourself, others, or life in general may be found through your own personal writings, in the silence of meditation, or in the symbolic states of both your dreams and your wakefulness. Such methods are discussed in the following chapter.

IV | We are all
orphans until we
find ourselves.

To Communicate With Oneself

Collective Creative Consciousness
Interconnectedness • Journal
Meditation • Dreams • Imagery
Traps

As a sculptor personally and meticu-
lously selects the appropriate tools
prior to merging with the virginal stone, so too self-help aids
are available from which the couple may choose to hone
their marriage and shape their pregnancy. Tools for
transformation would obviously vary with the uniqueness of
the couple. Pitfalls do exist, for it is easy to become intox-
icated by the narcissism of self-reflective methods or even
overcome by the responsibility of childbirth, but there is a
call for balance before conception.

Every creative act is preceded by some type of labor.
Pregnancy is a commitment to go within oneself and
beyond oneself; it has the potential to integrate individuals
into a family and the yet unborn into life.

Wholeness does not come from another person. Wholeness exists within. That exquisite moment of self-discovery,
of self-acceptance, of personal love, is invariably followed
within moments by the discovery of that same magnificence
within everyone and everything. To experience this
phenomenon is to know the link which unites all humanity.
The evolution of humankind toward wholeness is what the
great Hebraic philosopher Martin Buber refers to as the ebb
and flow of the individual from the "I-it" to the universal
"I-thou," which unites humankind. In the unification

process, it is as if wholeness seeks wholeness to create wholeness—the couple, as if in a hologram, unifies with another dimension of themselves and then integrates beyond themselves with their child. The synergy thus created in the merging of one human within another leads to the greatest love that we beings are capable of achieving.

Marriage, be it contractual or noncontractual, is a step towards entering that collective; that is, it is an attempt to be consciously part of more than oneself. The collective here does not mean an aggregate of human beings. We are talking of the formless collective *spirit* of consciousness that pervades all Being, an interrelationship that transcends persona, yet allows each person to maintain his or her identity. This is *the spirit of Interconnectedness.*

The collective consciousness is the sum total of the thoughts, acts and experiences of all life processes since the birth of creation itself. Your immortality is etched daily in its evolving memory disc. Think about the responsibility that your singular existence offers and also bathe in the joy of your gift received and your gift given. *You are part of the evolving collective consciousness called God.*

The newborn is the alchemic manifestation of such a union—the trinity that is born out of duality. The union of the mother and the father is greater than either of its parts. The creation and integration of this new form is the next step toward sharing in the extended collective. Each birth is a gift to the collective, yet also symbolically represents the price of admission.

So we see that the dyad created through marriage can evolve toward a triadic relationship. In a sense, the child can be considered as the third leg of a tripod, the leg that gives stability. But, in truth, each leg of the tripod is the third leg, each being equal and supportive of the other.

The friction within marriage can be born from the emotions that cause torque between inner searchings and outer realities associated with conception. These can expose the subtlest cracks in the armor that shields the couple's close but often vulnerable relationship. Still, this form of stress can also provide room for growth and rebirth of a marriage.

Stress, if understood, can serve as the prime mover in expanding the communion between couples, but if it is not appreciated as a potential gift, then it can further shatter an already fragile relationship. The intervals between thought and conception and conception and birth are the time to reassess the marriage and offer harmony as a gift to the shared creation—your child.

The experienced sailor appreciates the stress the wind creates as its force strikes the resistant sail. It is the resultant stress born of force and resistance that drives the yawing boat home. If, indeed, the wind should reach gale proportions, then the weathered sailor has the wisdom to furl the overpowered sails and ride the storm out. The sailor knows that, with patience and in time, he will continue his voyage, but only after the wind and sail work together once again in balanced harmony.

Health, life, love, and creation teeter on the fine edge of stress. Too little or too much leads to the pathological state of *dis*-stress. It is distress that sets the stage for mind/body *dis*-ease, not stress. Stress is more often than not the prime mover for transformation. This is the grace that is found within crisis, while distress is the chaotic, nondirected use of the same innate energy. Stress is responsible for humankind's movement and evolution. It can be a friend. Stress can serve as a stimulus to seek inner guidance and thus help one to obtain outer goals.

Even the most ideally conceived pregnancy is often associated with moments of doubt, bleakness, and anxiety; the distress is not only due to each prospective parent's struggle to maintain a singular identity, but each is continually driven by the child, as if in an offstage whisper, "Am I wanted? Are you prepared?" Demands placed upon the parents may wax and wane but, more often, continue to build in intensity throughout the pregnancy. The pain that often accompanies change can also be used to temper the creation before it is revealed in light and love.

Techniques are available by which we can learn to communicate more effectively with ourselves, with others, and as a couple. These self-directed techniques can enhance inner growth and understanding and provide creative change. One such method to enhance self-interaction is journal-keeping as described by Ira Progoff in his book *At a Journal Workshop*. A diary allows one to work and play with both the joys and the sorrows of one's interpersonal relationships and past experiences. By carrying on various dialogues (through writing) with those people who touch our lives, in whatever manner, or even with those events which have affected our health or choice of career, we can begin to understand more clearly our unique path through life.

It is after such soul-searching, carried out through writing and reflection, that our newly found understanding can point the way for active transformation. By active transformation, I mean we become co-creators with the stimuli of our environment rather than bystanders who are buffeted about by the circumstances of life. We can actively evolve and thus prepare more fully for parenthood and/or adulthood.

The language of everyday conversation often bypasses the wisdom of our thoughts. The written word is a truer representation of thought and can be repeatedly used for reflective problem solving. The more rapidly we are able to write our thoughts, the truer becomes our perception of the wisdom of the unconscious. In a *personal* journal, we can speak uninhibitedly to the silent adversary with whom we may share the paradoxes of emotions such as love and pain or hopefulness and helplessness. We can assume all the roles of those individuals with whom communication is needed, as well as contact the child or mother and father within that craves rebirth. This time the adult can review the past events or the child within through a less judgmental perspective. To imagine assuming another's role, a past personal role, or even an unexperienced one in the quiet, safe place of a diary is comparable to the American Indian adage, "Walk in my moccasins before you judge me."

The impersonality of expressing thoughts and emotions on paper can offer greater insight into what previously appeared to be unresolvable problems, problems with family, friends, self, or even work. Difficulties created through the unfinished business of the past can jaundice decision making in the present.

The diary should be kept private. It is only for you; therefore, it should remain discreet. These directives enhance the uninhibited flow of your writing. The moment there is the urge to share your insights with another, the more sequestered the unconscious flow becomes as it hides from the ego. This is in contradistinction to the dream state in which the unconscious rules. The value of the unobstructed wisdom of the unconscious can only be judged by you and by the transformations that follow within your life. As thought is transmuted into the matrix of the written word, so, too, will the matrix of your relationship change within your work and your communication with others. You are preparing not only for the birth of another but for a rebirth of yourself into health.

Healing can take place through a diary dialogue. Disease is the transformational process of a body that can no longer wait for the mind to initiate change. It is as if the mind said to the body, "Begin without me." While on the other hand, mental illness is a mind in transformation that is housed in a stagnant body—nobody is home. Healing is the transformational process towards mind-body integration. Spirit is always integrated but we tend to be blind to it except in the rare instances of balance.

A diary may unlock dark emotions and tap the wisdom of your Inner Teacher—your soul that waits to be heard—the voice that eviscerates your struggle and gives you direction. The light of understanding shed on a memory distorted through time can transmute disharmony to harmony like ice to cool clear water. Journal-keeping can awaken that Inner Teacher, who clearly points out those paths to take and those to avoid. It is in the transcending of this dark side of your conflicts that you are more often likely to reflect the light of understanding that is so essential for initiating transformation.

If we run only towards the sun, we never experience the trailing shadow. Often to bring more brightness into our personal universe and that of others, it is essential that we stop, turn and face the darkness and so carry light into our fears. It is especially for this reason that the terms "disharmony" and "harmony" are used rather than "correct" and "incorrect," "right" or "wrong." Such words carry with them implicit judgment, comparison, and guilt.

Harmony and disharmony are relative terms and not pure states. Truth, happiness and love are probably balanced somewhere in between these two conditions, but occupy such a fine, yet changeable point in time/space that it is difficult to know when you're there. However, it is all too obvious when you are not, and you find yourself thrust into the desolation of disharmony. This discomfort gives you the energy to shift awareness towards center, towards harmony. Disharmony is initially resolved through understanding and completed through change. Disharmony is the stimulus for change and a source of creativity. Disharmony has a fluidity about it as compared to the solid destructive state of "wrong." (The music of Stravinsky was considered dissonant by the critics only until it was understood.) Therefore, the conscious or unconscious disharmony that appears as discord and clouds intimate relationships can always be shifted towards harmony by a new accord. I am reminded of my most favorite childhood radio program— *The Shadow*—"Who knows . . . the Shadow knows."

But beware! Don't go into the shadow alone on an overcast day. Illness or depression can cause a loss of discernment and so an illusion of unfathomable despair. On such desperate days questions are typically asked too late and answers are typically too contrived. We are like computers: put garbage in—you'll get garbage out. In times of prolonged suffering a friend or therapist can serve you as a guide, a mirror that offers you the needed balance to find clarity. However, a sunny day, a day filled with understanding, is the time to engage those shadowed fears alone. In a literal sense, if you stand under the sun, the margins of your shadow become clearly stencilled and grounded. The sun-filled day awaits your indulgence and offers you self-knowledge. You are both the light and the dark. Both aspects offer gifts for growth. To accept your shadow is to accept your humanness and so to learn compassion. How can you judge another when you are the totality of all things? To judge another is to judge yourself.

Perhaps someday we will no longer need to use anxiety, illness, or challenge as the prime mover for transformation. However, until that time, disharmony should be honored as being essential for personal and collective growth. Prolonged bliss, created either through force without resistance or security without change, is a stalemate. Such bliss is death to the creative process. In the future, as individuals realize that they can survive the risk of change and experience that nothing is lost in the act of transformation, then change will be voluntarily sought. At that time in history, the universal prod of discomfort will be replaced by the more subtle act of love as the initiator for transformation and voluntary service.

Harmony is not bliss. Harmony is balance. It, too, can lead to a disquietness. We often feel so stable that we can't stand it, so we create problems to recreate a more familiar base state. Harmony can shift towards disharmony as an act of creation. Harmony and disharmony, as is true for most opposites, are relative states of each other, yet the interplay between the two serves as a major source of the transformational process. Journal-keeping offers insights into this creative process and at the same time provides understanding into one's interpersonal relationships, one's work and one's body.

Meditation can be another method for self-discovery, decision making, or change. Meditation is useful in the self-regulation of disharmony and harmony through the release of natural tranquilizing substances within the body. Since the brain has the ability to produce chemicals capable of creating the appropriate emotional response to a given stimulus such as hunger, anger, fear, or tranquility, then perhaps these responses can be self-regulated. Most therapeutic drugs work either through blocking these specific substances or by increasing the duration or quantity of their release. It has been recently demonstrated that morphine does not cause pain relief per se; this drug affects the brain's release of endorphins—pain killers. Therefore, morphine is a computerized punch card that triggers the brain computer to release its own chemical opiate.

A placebo (a substance given as medicine but which has no therapeutic value) can afford relief for approximately 35 percent of patients who have pain. In the past, these patients were often chastised and cast aside as hypochondriacs. However, recent research has shown that if a drug is given to block the self-produced brain opiate, then those individuals who would normally respond to the administration of the placebo will experience pain. Therefore, physiologically and psychologically, these individuals had been able to control the chemistry of their minds. Previously, we physicians discharged these gifted people as "crocks," and forfeited the opportunity to study self-healers and thereby enhance our own medical knowledge. If we had studied the mechanisms by which these "malingerers," who refer to physicians as "quacks," were able to control their own biochemistry, we could have been further along the path of a drug-free society. We could also have resolved the "crock-quack" syndrome!

Other opiates, tranquilizers, and hallucinogens all can be found in the brain waiting to be controlled naturally. Future therapy may lie not so much in drug pharmacology as in the power of the will to selectively release these factors. The drug of the future may be self-directed will power with a coherency, intensity, and single-mindedness of purpose similar to a laser.

Indian fakirs and yogis, who in meditation regulate the physiology of their hearts and their threshold to pain, demonstrate what can be achieved through self-directed thought. Meditation may work through the self-regulation of the chemistry of the brain, which has the power to mediate the heart rate and, at the same time, release appropriate substances to decrease pain and promote healing. It is not necessary to be from the Far East to program similar directives into your own bio-computer—holographic mind.

One way I learned meditation was by watching potato bugs, turtles, and snails. When the external world threatens these creatures, they retreat and retract inwardly. Just so, in silence we can transcend life's confusions by going into ourselves. In such a state, complexities become simplified, and orderly options come into focus. The Zen metaphor for meditation which tells of dipping a bucket into one's well and then slowly partaking of the water is a fitting one. The deep water that supplies one spring supplies all wells. When we tap The Source, we tap all sources and obtain universal truth and knowledge. We can learn from the smallest of creatures to the wisest of men that often the best method to resolve stress is not to seek outside oneself for ways to conquer pain, isolation, and suffering, but to go within.

In Shimon Halevi's book, *The Way of Kabbalah,* he writes, "In order to rise up Jacob's ladder of the road of the universe, one must descend into the depths of one's own being. Here we see a simultaneous inner and outer movement, with the microcosm of man reflecting the macrocosm of the manifest world."

He speaks to the contraction and relaxation phase that precedes all acts of creation. But in meditation it is specifically the labor of the unconscious self or perhaps the collective consciousness that Pierre Teilhard de Chardin speaks of that seeks recognition. In that inner movement of intuitive exchange one is outwardly reborn.

The application of intuition is creation. The insightful person can now reach out and expand beyond self to embrace others. The discreet margins that separate individuals are blurred. This places the meditator, the person of focused singular thoughts, at the threshold of a dream, at the edge of an extended reality, and so within the reach of the collective consciousness. The meditator is inseparable from all existence.

Meditation is a method by which we can enter this state and sift through the different options available to simplify life's apparent confusions. I would like to share my personal form of meditation with you. Meditation is point focus, so first find a place of quiet to stand, sit, or lie down and, most importantly, to become silent. Gently close your eyes and place your hands in the prayer position, approximately twelve inches in front of your face. As slowly as possible, separate your hands, micrometer by micrometer, and in your mind's eye think only of the space between your separating hands. The point of focus is space. Space is infinite and gently guides you into the "oneness" of the collective, the place of unification. Continue to keep your eyes closed, moving your hands as slowly as possible in cadence with your breathing. You will notice a slight increase in hand separation on inhalation and a coming together on expiration. Experience the quality of space between your hands or the color projections that emanate from your mind. Experience all five senses of the silent life. After a variable period of time, slowly turn the palms of your hands up and as slowly as possible allow them to descend softly upon the tops of your thighs. When the backs of your hands touch your thighs, relax your shoulders, yet continue to be aware of the rhythm of your breathing, or for that matter, anything that comes into your consciousness. You may hear the sound of a plane overhead, the rustling leaves of a tree, or the sound of music. Integrate all the sounds and thoughts of that moment into your being but also allow them to flow through you uninterrupted. Soon, you become the plane, the tree, the music. There is no separation between you, your thoughts, or the outside world. You *are* the meditation, the meditation is you. To complete the meditative cycle, simply return your hands to the prayer position and slowly open your eyes. Notice the vibrance of the room. Touch the chair or feel the carpet. Smell the room's scent and taste its essence. Hear life!

Over a period of time, as you lose the discernment between the inner world of meditation and the outer world of "reality," life itself becomes the mantra—the point of focus of the meditation. Now, with your eyes wide open, you can enter the plane of active meditation—life. All those pleasant, sensual, physiological experiences that have been programmed into your mind and body during that quiet meditative state can now be carried into the activities of your daily life.

For thousands of years, wise men have suggested various methods to achieve inner peace. The simple, rhythmic repetition of a single word, act, or thought (mantra) has the ability to quiet the constant chatting of our minds. This is aptly referred to in Eastern philosophy as the "monkey's mind." Therefore, meditation is a perfect teacher of the art of maintaining the pure intention needed for parenthood. Single-mindedness of thought can penetrate the confusion produced during decision making. Logical priorities can be formulated in meditative silence. As in journal keeping, the Inner Teacher can be touched. I wonder if this is the rationale which causes Eastern philosophers to state, "See through a single eye," or the Judaic directive, "They (God's words) should be held for frontlets between thine eyes." Meditation is a silent prayer that can be carried into the day's activities. It involves point concentration upon a singular thought carried out in any atmosphere. The meditative methods are only for beginners; for the experienced meditator there are no methods. Life itself becomes the meditation.

A portion of any meditation can also be devoted to the mantra of love and directed to a family member, friend, or acquaintance. A positive singular thought or affirmation can be programmed into the timelessness of any meditation. The point of balance that exists between the wakefulness yet somnolence of the trance-like state of meditation is fertile for reprogramming one's life and communicating beyond words with others. Itzhak Bentov, in his book *Stalking the Wild Pendulum,* refers to this timeless state as "zero rest." This state is similar to what the physicists refer to as "ground state."

This timeless phase is a point of total potentiality. Rene Thom, in his "Catastrophe Theory," hypothesizes that in the moment of timelessness when the equilibrium between two discontinuous and divergent phenomena breaks down, change and transformation occur. It is precisely during such a still point that the less preoccupied creatures of earth (cockroaches, ants, and other things that creep) forecast earthquakes. Phylogenetically, we have buried within us the same awareness, the same potentiality, and the same knowing that quakes in its labor to be born.

The initial, passive, receptive form of meditation sets the stage for an inner equilibrium and integration to occur. The secondary, active, directed form of meditation contains affirmations or projections for self and others and thereby has the force to disrupt the moment of timelessness. This disruption raises the scaffolding for personal transformation. The integration of both the active and the passive forms of meditation lead to repeated consciousness tremors. Therefore, we see that stillness followed by pure intent allows for creative change. There are then two varying yet complementary forms of meditation at work. The first allows us *to be* while the second allows us *to become*.

The choice of a method for meditation depends upon the uniqueness and discernment of the individuals involved. Awareness, like understanding and happiness, is something you give yourself. They cannot be given away, bought, or sold.

Many disciples of self-awareness meditation groups are often drawn to the light of their teacher as a moth to a bright bulb, but all too often the devotees become blinded by the guru's radiance and, like the moth, can be singed. The guru closest to you is often you. The power of Reverend Jones and the mass suicide of his 900 devotees attests to the truth of this statement. The tragedy in Guyana is a severe yet valuable teacher for "the new age consciousness movement" to become fully awake. The lesson to be learned is: to surrender within the collective does not mean to lose oneself or give up one's choice.

Before individuals are allowed to walk within your mind they should take off their shoes. By this, I mean that helpers should wait for the helpee to ask for help. The helper should then ask permission of himself through meditation, as to whether he should or should not enter the contract. The mind is the temple of the soul and so the visitor should humbly bow as a token for the gift of entry. This is informed consent, be it between a teacher and a student, a physician and a patient, or a wife and a husband.

Meditative techniques, like prescribed chemical tranquilizers, can become addictive. The formless world of meditation offers succor from the everyday obstacles and problems of life. Although meditation may seem to be innocuous, it, too, has its own traps.

In the quest for the ecstasy of personal and spiritual enlightenment, we often lose sense of the common ground we share with humanity, a ground of being present, of being totally here. Maybe this is true because we seek *E-c-s-t-a-s-y*. A case in point is the woman who came to me exasperated by her alcoholic husband and his total intolerance of her "all too frequent meditations." But, in talking it out, she soon realized his need for alcohol was usually set off by circumstances similar to those that drove her to seek solace in meditation. Each partner was using his and her own form of escape. Meditation should not be utilized as a shield to block or even relieve one's anxieties. *Meditation is not medication.* Meditation, like all things in life, is a question of balance.

Our lives are not an either/or existence. Humankind's task is to live in two worlds simultaneously—the hard structured world of "reality" can be juxtaposed and integrated with the soft, formless collective world of intuition. These worlds are not separate, but each is an extension of the other. Carlos Castaneda refers to these worlds as the "nigual," the formless, and the "tonal," the formed. They are not mutually exclusive, but can merge harmoniously with each other. This split, yet unified, perception of life is symbolically and figuratively represented by the intuitive right and the deductive left hemispheres of the brain. When these dualistic aspects are so inexorably entwined that they co-exist in harmony, then the ultimate state of balance is achieved. This is the state of total wakefulness.

To me, total wakefulness is equivalent to balanced schizophrenia. This is the state in which the formless is integrated into the form of everyday living. Wakefulness is the point of integration that occurs when the mirror images of form and formlessness come into a singular focus. To function only within a singular *non*integrated hemisphere of the brain is like taking a shower with a raincoat. To find the balance in all things, is to come home to the center of personal understanding. The Taoist calls this "the still point." It is when the body and mind co-exist in harmony that we evolve the spirit. Spirit is always there. Spirit is balance itself and in that exquisite moment of balance the individual moves with the collective in a singular wave along the infinite spiral of life. In that moment of mind and body interaction, duality is found to be but an illusion.

Dreams, too, are as much a part of our existence as is the waking state. In the closing of eyes during meditation, relaxation, or sleep, the incoming stimuli are diminished, and the inner world is the focal point. Like a child who places a blanket over her head and asks profoundly, "Where did everyone go?" perhaps the darkness rekindles the child's memory and desire for rebirth—the ultimate game of life.

It is also during sleep that our intellect, our ego, steps aside and allows uncluttered thoughts to travel unprocessed through our consciousness. In sleep, the past and the present events of wakefulness are sorted out and filed symbolically. The computerized holographic mind, through symbolism, rearranges the information in what appears to be a totally illogical manner to the rational brain. The mind is neither the brain nor the intellect. The mind is the synthesizer of our life experience and if we are wise enough to pay attention, it is director. But the often bizarre symbols produced during the dream state allow the drama to continue without interruption. In fact, if we had full understanding of what was being projected in the moment of dreaming, we would either block it, cancel it, or still worse, interrupt it with our logical orchestrations. In fact, we often do this by suddenly awakening in the middle of the night. This is no more than a gesture of "Stop the world, I want to get off. I no longer want to see, feel, or hear any more of *that* scenario!"

Our dreams are valid reflections of our composite life experiences and also provide precognitive insights into the future. And so, dreams can offer wise solutions for emotional blocks or indecisions. To share your dreams with another or to write them down or even to meditate upon their symbolism will often unmask the deeper yet higher meaning of those visionary states. A spouse, lover, or friend can be an excellent mirror to reflect upon your dreams. Such sharing may assist you in your choice of whether to conceive or not to conceive. However, whether you explore your dreams using the symbols as described by Freud or Jung, or even with the counsel of a dream therapist, the final interpretations and their application is up to you. Innumerable books and methods are available to assist you in dream analysis. If this method of self-discovery appeals to you, explore it.

As in meditation, there are active and passive dream states; both are gifts. As an example, before going to sleep, while in that twilight state that is identical to the trance-like state of meditation, ask yourself a question and then dream the answer. If the answer does not come, graciously accept the wisdom that replaced it. The phase just prior to being fully awake also provides a similar interface for altered (out of the ordinary) yet prophetic states of consciousness. Perhaps all dreams are not worth remembering or even worth reporting. But you cannot forget the dream of prophecy, the dream of dreams. You may also be assured that many of your forgotten dreams consciously return as a barrage of creative thoughts that fill your mind in the shower, during your breakfast, or even during your drive to work. Although these thoughts were conceived as symbols during the night's repose, they are often subtly brought into form by your actions. *Awakening can be an awakening.*

However, please don't complicate your dreams by over-analysis. The lack of drama of your midnight movie might not raise your interest, but some of the deepest insights come from looking at the ordinary in a different way. Just think how well our intellect can botch things. The intellect more often than not distorts even the perceptions of our waking state. If it weren't for the intellect getting in the way, we would appreciate how the symbols of everyday living that stimulate our five senses (be they birds, planes, smells, music, the sway of a tree, the taste of a kiss, or the touch of the wind) are also recorded in our brain. These apparently mundane perceptions are as symbolic as the guide-posts in our dreams. Every moment of breath is significant and symbolic.

Unconscious dreams are as much a part of conscious life as is conscious life of unconscious dreams. Dreams are a significant part of life and as such continue to unfold, revealing their true nature at a later date.

Mental imagery, or waking dream states, is another method for choosing options. It has become reasonably well established that imagery and ordinary perception seem, in effect, to be manifestations of a common brain process. In brief, a human's visual perceptions as well as fantasies are not only the gate to consciousness but subserve the unconscious. If, as Dr. Robert Livingston, a noted neurologist, states, reality and imagination share common pathways and access roots within the brain, then fantasy can a be painless preparation for reality. Fantasy can also create a most painful reality. Step right up—pay your money—make your choice. Imagery has been used by athletes to enhance their performance, and more recently, Dr. Carl Simonton has used imagery as part of his treatment for the cancer patient. Is it necessary to have either a goal in life or an illness in order to program one's life more fortuitously?

By looking ahead, the entire pregnancy, delivery, post-partum period, and even the adulthood of the child can be projected on the three-dimensional screen of the couple's minds. Even this fanciful experience could make the choice of whether or not to conceive more relevant. Each phase of the prenatal, birth, and post-partum periods will be found to offer its own unique challenge. Potential parents can visualize themselves in each of these time frames. In fact, the entire pregnancy can be played out in thought forms or acted out in psychodrama before being consumated.

The unconscious, whether expressed through writing, dreams, meditation, or imagery, is free to express life fully and in its own terms through the language of spontaneous symbols. When we can be as consciously accepting as our unconscious, we can assume more responsibility for the present and a purer love can take form. At that time, the question of whether to enter pregnancy or not is no longer burdensome. Choice is an act of grace. I often wonder if we are not totally asleep, swimming in a sea of unconsciousness, occasionally gasping in moments of deep inspiration. For some, an inspiring thought would also be that love and creativity can be more permanently expressed by a decision not to have a child at all.

The shattering of old belief systems that often results from self-analysis is the seed for new beginnings. All the tools for self-discovery, such as hypnosis, rebirthing, psychotherapy, meditation, journal keeping, dreams, or whatever, are available, but the choice of the most efficacious method can only be decided by you. It takes work to search out your specific path and your specific method, but the effort can prepare you for the patterning of future generations. If a technique does not work for you, it does not negate its value for others, or for that matter, even for yourself at another time. Perhaps your metaphor is dance, art or music. In either case, let it be, let you be. Your uniqueness is your Gift to Life.

New methods for consciousness awakening are being developed daily, many are identical in nature to methods of old, yet all have an intrinsic worth. Each new exploration can serve as fertile ground upon which individual growth can take place. The method chosen, however, should subserve the individual who, in turn, will convert it into his or her own personal form. The method should return the individual to himself or herself. The individual should not be a clone for the method. For if this occurs, then the self becomes lost and with it the reason for being—creative transformation. Methods, like people, can become false gods and eventually, as clay idols, must be put aside in order that personal uninhibited growth can take place. It is your unique transformation which is the gift that you bequeath to all children.

Life is like the petri dish that is filled with a nutrient broth and is used to culture bacteria. Society, parents, family, friends, and lovers, as well as all the various new age methods for actualization, are no more than teachers who streak your culture medium. What grows is more than either its ingredients or its contributors. What emerges is *you.*

There is an old Chinese proverb: "Don't paint as the masters painted, but see what the masters saw." In reality, a new method is usually one that is presented in either a new jargon or one which penetrates your resistant consciousness. The method works because it recalls something already present within you. We can only understand what we already know. Therefore, give some of the credit to yourself. An unknown author once wrote:

"You cannot be given a life by someone else. Of all the people you will know in a lifetime, you are the only one you will never leave or lose. To the question of your life, you are the only answer. To the problems of your life, you are the only solution."

In order to convert our unconsciousness to consciousness or thought to form, we must find within ourselves the catalyst for self-knowledge—understanding. Once we surrender to the Inner Teacher which patiently awaits within each one of us, we can begin to control our own personal lives and co-create the universe with others. But, more importantly, we can learn to communicate more effectively with other beings who are but our mirrored reflections.

C. G. Jung said, "The Self is a circle whose center is everywhere and whose circumference is nowhere." We are all orphans until we find that self. The self is synonymous with The Inner Teacher, The Soul, or that essence of Godly love which is within each one of us. This is what is truly meant by "coming home." When the Self is acknowledged, each prospective parent has finished his or her preparation for the question to conceive or not to conceive and is better equipped for the pregnant interval.

There is a labor that even precedes conception and is essential for life. It is the labor of inner work. The quality of that work is not only reflected in the quality of our creations but in the quality of all existence. Our labor is our gift to eternal life.

V

Pregnancy is not
only the birth of
a new physical
form, but the test
of a marriage.

The Pregnant Interval

Relationships • Games People Play
Romance • Love • Service

T he sculptor's chisel has been set. The forceful blow meets the resistant stone and in the moment of impact, the creative act has been initiated. The momentous interval between thought and manifestation has begun. The sculpture begins to take form. The philosopher Bertrand Russell says it another way: "It is the interval between notes that creates the music—not the notes themselves."

Although pregnancy is defined as that period of time between conception and birth, it is more. Pregnancy, as stated previously, begins in thought. If that thought is to give birth to life, then life in turn carries the intention of pregnancy. Life now becomes a never-ending continuum of repeated births into an unfolding life. The tapestry of life is patterned in pregnancy.

If the thought of pregnancy precedes fertilization and continues as thought beyond birth, then pregnancy is but a slice of life that gives life to life. Conception and delivery are merely points in time that give spice to life and as such are too often confused with being the *sine qua non* of pregnancy.

The nine-month gestation period called pregnancy is a time capsule that holds within it all the ingredients that are found in life itself. These months are filled with conditions and contracts, joys and sorrow, pain and pleasures. The pregnant interval is also a time to learn patience and compassion, surrender and trust, tolerance and praise, knowledge and understanding, and finally, the sum of all its parts—love. Pregnancy is a teacher of life.

The newborn is conceived in that moment appropriately referred to as "making love"—a moment when formless love is made into manifest love. The subsequent nine months can cloud that moment and warp the greatest of all intentions—making love—so that the focused thought of love is often dulled by the day-to-day tasks needed to maintain many of our other previous creations: marriage, work, home, and hobbies. While pregnancy may offer many moments of exhilaration and excitement, there can be equal periods of frustration and isolation. If pregnancy encompasses all the drama of a complete lifetime, it, too, offers a test to the mariage, a test that can either temper a relationship between man and woman or fracture it.

The nine-month gestation period should provide adequate time for stabilization of the marriage. The nine-month interval is a period when the couple can transcend society's longheld opinion that pregnancy is just a consequence and logical sequence of marriage. This is a time to work through the new realities of an old relationship with both one's partner and with oneself in order to prepare for the intrusion of something new. This is not only true for the first-born but for all subsequent pregnancies. Intrusion may seem to be a harsh word, but a child, as any creation or work of art, changes all that preceded it.

Doctor Leon Israel stated, at the Sex Information and Education Council of the United States in 1967, that ". . . a problem between the two people is not usually resolved by the addition of a third person. On the contrary, the third person may disrupt a formerly adequate relationship of the original pair."

In spite of this, the affirmation by the doctor that the pregnancy does indeed exist is usually greeted with explosive joy on the part of the couple who craves this child. The news often resolves a previously deep-seated doubt: "Can we have children?" The moment also heralds a potential change in the societal roles of husband and wife to that of father and mother. But this shift is only partially true. Roles are not necessarily exchanged in the creative process. In fact, the relationships that co-exist between husband and wife and mother and father provide the couple with perhaps their newest and greatest challenge for growth.

Life is not an either/or or win/lose ball game. It is compromise. To the Taoist this is known as the Tao, the path, the point of integrated paradoxes, the "still point." It is not a dull, bland place but a point of dynamic movement. The dynamic interchange at the center of paradoxes or opposites is so rapid that it only appears still. On a simpler level it can be experienced in the child's game of seesaw. Movement stops only when either side of the plank becomes overweighted. Dynamic, yet unsettled, movement is necessary to maintain that fine point of balance which keeps both players elevated and level. Pregnancy presents a true test of the couple's willingness to balance, elevate, and integrate their multiple and paradoxical relationships of life.

The disparate male and female energies come into play early in the first stage of pregnancy as the husband internalizes "I did it," but his "I-ness" is balanced by her "I got it," "mine-ness." The expectant mother experiences sensations ranging from nausea to feelings of bliss. It is nearly impossible for the expectant father to relate to "her pregnancy" or to keep pace with the wild variations of her mood swings. He does not see any outward change in his wife's condition and often questions whether the positive pregnancy test might not belong to another. (Sporadically, throughout the pregnancy, they may both wish it did.) But for now, there is no question in the mind of the mother-to-be: "I am with child." She knows not only that the pregnancy exists, but that she is completely and intimately pregnant. During this phase, the expectant father is often prone to feelings of rejection and uselessness, yet, paradoxically, he may also feel an urgency to prepare both economically and morally for the event. Under this self-imposed pressure, he tends to work harder at his job, becomes more frugal, and, at the same time, seeks to be closer to his wife.

The husband now becomes the archetypal provider, "the bread winner." This need reflects more an insecurity about not being an active part of the unfolding embryo than the need to provide. The husband tends to match and compare his external endeavors to his wife's internal creation—"that's her job; this is mine." There is a disconnectedness, a disassociation from the unity that is represented by the pregnancy.

It is a given fact that women carry the formed pregnancy, but it is not so well known or even accepted that men, too, are pregnant but bear the silent formless pregnancy. Pregnancy is co-creation, co-transformation. To compare contributions is absurd. The frustration that some men and fewer women act out in response to not experiencing the total pregnancy is not only destructive but is the absurdity itself.

It is of interest to me that those women who have delivered a child do not in any way lose a desire to create through another medium such as work, but they do lose an obsessive *need* to create. Perhaps if men could touch, for but a moment, the formless inner essence of creation itself, then they might have less of a need to prove themselves to themselves and others by creating from outside themselves. This relentless striving to prove to oneself and others may be the source of man's inhumanity to man. Although it is precisely this striving that brings about culture, art, civilization, and evolution, we must learn how to channel and use our passion less destructively.

Love and caring in our society are too often measured by the frequency of making love. Nevertheless, Masters and Johnson have described the first trimester (the first three months of pregnancy) as a time of decreased coital interest for women. This variance in sexual needs might be brought about by the dramatic physiologic changes that occur during this time. There may be breast tenderness, nausea, fatigue, and a decrease in vaginal secretions. During this time, if there is a lack of communication, understanding, and patience, coupled with a feeling of isolation, then the father-to-be is likely to interpret his personal experience as rejection. This dis-tress of pregnancy can often lead the husband or the wife to that first extramarital encounter.

Extramarital relationships often bring with them an unrelenting guilt. To assuage this pain, the husband or wife may justify their disharmony by telling themselves they are married not only to the wrong person, but that they are inexorably trapped by the pregnancy. Justification is too often indignant self-rationalization which allows us to do whatever we wanted to do. Such rationalization often further deepens the isolation, which is mirrored as a rejection. And still, no one talks! This experience is just as common for a couple in a noncontractual free "marriage," only now the child becomes the contract and represents all they had attempted to avoid by not entering a traditional marriage—attachment. Any future disharmony between the couple is often displaced incorrectly on "that child."

Another example of diffused energy is the mother-to-be who seeks compensation for her outer loneliness by overly integrating with the pregnancy, and thus her relationship becomes an intramarital one, but, in this case, with the unborn. The contentment and security of this internalized relationship (for the wife) can extend beyond labor and delivery and into the child's adulthood. The gain of one family member may be bought with the loss of another—its father. Following the delivery, the reverse may occur in the father's moment of attachment when he sees *"his"* child for the first time and screams in silence: "My God, *she was pregnant!"*

The pregnant woman is also faced with her own fears of inadequacy concerning motherhood. She may feel completely unprepared for the formidable prospect of having her own child. She questions: Were her explorations at playing house as a child sufficient schooling for this task? Does babysitting provide enough education for a degree in parenting? Is her pelvis adequate? Can she spiritually nurture the newborn? These are common fears. The husband, the wife, and all of society expect the pregnant woman to have inherent qualities of motherhood which, when appropriately stimulated by the mere fact of conception, miraculously flourish and flower.

When under stress, the prospective parents should tap their own deeper essence and seek to know and to feel their partner's needs. If this is not accomplished, then each may remain oblivious to the other's frustrations, which by now may be expressed in that extramarital relationship, in becoming a workaholic, or in becoming disenchanted with the unborn child. The energy generated through stress is too often dissipated, as the hole in the balloon that prevents its ascension. The "apparently" negative influences of the coping ego are lost as a "potential" liberator for creative change. Positive and negative are relative aspects of the same force; both are transformational. The final outcome of their use is always left to the individual.

Even the most stable relationship can become tenuous if conception has been preceded by a history of infertility or a miscarriage. Under these circumstances, legitimate fear may be superimposed upon the pregnancy. The wife and husband may be justifiably worried about another pregnancy. This fear is often acted out by the couple who, during love making, are overly concerned about disrupting the pregnancy. "High risk" pregnancies can put a strain on a marriage to a far greater degree than would be expected for the couple embarking upon a first pregnancy or the couple whose prior pregnancy was uncomplicated.

A case in point was that of a couple who had great difficulty in conceiving. When at last they became pregnant, the husband, both in love and in fear, refrained from intercourse for the entire nine months. He was preoccupied by his desire to preserve the pregnancy. He played tennis for two to three hours a day as an emotional escape and rationalized the generalized avoidance of his wife as caused by fatigue. He even increased his working hours and assumed outside projects which he would normally never have undertaken. Communication was nonexistent.

Naturally, yet inappropriately, his wife misinterpreted his "coolness" as a result of her "gross, inept, and unappealing body." She, in turn, responded with depression and fatigue.

Their mutual isolation furthered their lack of communication. This distancing became the familiar pattern and was carried into the birth and beyond. The unresolved misinterpretation of love was the seed for the new unproductive relationship. Before the child's second birthday, the marriage ended, predictably, in divorce.

The history of this couple is typical and represents a breakdown of communication, both verbal and nonverbal, that frequently occurs during pregnancy. If neither partner makes an attempt to assuage anxieties by confronting his or her fears, either through talking them out or through inner confrontation, then a potentially creative form of energy becomes dissipated through avoidance.

The wife's depression, fatigue, and isolation were a reflected image of her husband's. She absorbed the misinterpretation and assumed it as her own. She lost her identity and became the universal sponge and so became the self-fulfilled prophecy: "gross, inept, and unappealing." Since the two avoided any attempt to use their common pain as a source for renewal, the relationship ended. The only things shared in this pregnancy were their depression, fatigue, and isolation.

The memory set for despair and rejection was well ingrained within nine months. The two sought to resolve their unfinished business outside of themselves and through encounters with other mates. Little did they realize that personal unfinished business cannot be resolved by another. In fact, to bring the loose threads of a tattered garment into another is adulterous to the new cloth. It is patchwork.

People can resolve their conflicts in love. In so doing, they have the option either to stay in love or leave in love. Such relationships set the stage for either the continuation of an unencumbered present or an entirely new beginning.

Another potential for trouble and/or transformation awaits those couples who have been married for many years but who have delayed their pregnancy until one partner has obtained a post-post-doctorate degree while the other partner worked to assure financial security. Now, more than ever, they need to communicate and share thoughts and feelings. People who have been married for two or more years usually seem to adjust with greater ease to new situations such as pregnancy. However, problems often arise when their needs become so interconnected that their individual identity is lost. Too often the pregnancy, and later the child, become an intrusion into their fused relationship. The unborn child demands to be included in what was once the parents' world of security and oneness, and he or she offers the relationship an option for further growth.

If a husband or wife experienced isolation prior to conception, there is always the possibility that these former feelings can be rekindled and enhanced by the first sign of separation that the pregnancy may cause. If the *emotional* computer/holographic mind prints out a distillation of all previous, similar feelings such as separation, loneliness, and rejection, then the personal pain becomes out of proportion to the immediate situation. It is clear that the nine-month period is long enough to either burn out or reprogram the prospective parents' computers.

It is implicit in most of the Eastern and Western philosophies that a person is a totality of all of his or her experiences. The maze of complexities that escapes awareness as we tiptoe through life can often become overwhelming. It is only after being awakened by an emotional shock or illness that we exclaim "Why me?" or "Poor me!" If we had taken the risk of stepping on but a few of life's thorns perhaps we would have been better prepared for the answer.

These points (pun not intended) are not presented to sell fear but to alert the reader to the dynamics which can destroy marriage and the family and might set the stage for chronic disease. The understanding of marriage, family, and dishealth was taught to me as a result of the wisdom that many of my friends gained through their insights into their own illnesses.

Emotionally and physiologically, chronic illness, as the birthing process, unfolds so gradually that family members are often ignorant of the distance that has come between them. This disparity is precisely why communication becomes so difficult, yet why communication is so essential for bonding. Although paths should be united by illness and birth, unification is not without labor. In such circumstances, no one speaks to the issues of feelings, emotions, and needs. There is a shield of silence that is occasionally penetrated by small talk. Salvation is occasionally grasped through the eternal hope that the pervading cloud of disquiet will pass. Why is so much more found to be said after death or divorce?

Pregnancy is not illness, although doctors, family, and society often react to it as such. Pregnancy symbolically must be seen as an extension beyond self and towards others in health. Cancer and mental illness will also someday be understood to be the body's or mind's abortive attempt to break through to a healthier state of being. Cancer is the illness of our time and is a perfect metaphor for a transformational society that is crying desparately for change even it if means death to some viable institutions.

Even during the stress of a highly charged experience, be it illness or divorce, physicians, family and friends, in their attempts to block the pain or stop the person from escaping to an egoless reality, often freeze the individual in his or her phobia. This is done through *too much* support, psychotropic drugs, shock therapy and, yes, even psychotherapy. Perhaps the psychotic-like state should be accepted as a transitional one that can lead, through supportive love, to a new balance, to a new octave of experiencing life. Can we sit patiently while someone experiences either discomfort or a different reality than societal consensus? Can we be present enough to hug without holding?

Many books were written in the '70s about the need for personal space. But the truth is we cohabit space. Actually, "them out there" is "us in here." We are a dynamic, expanding, boundless, yet interconnected community of humankind motivated to evolve consciousness. Through the acceptance of cohabitation there is neither the loss of self nor the loss of one's personal freedom, but the awareness that each individual permanently impacts all members of the community.

Pregnancy can be either the battleground or the training field to begin the scaffolding for a new quantum of Collective Creative Consciousness. Pregnancy is but one of the many ways to learn about such an evolving community.

Even the isolated nuclear family is being shattered into the atomic family. To relieve the isolation that such lonely people feel as a result of either a divorce, illness, retirement, death of a loved one, or pregnancy, the extended family or community is being created. These communities are often conceived in loneliness and bonded by the matrix of a common need. These communities often begin as singles groups for the divorced, *make today count* groups for the cancer person, retirement groups for the aged, bereavement groups for survivors, meditation groups for the seekers, and childbirth preparation classes for the pregnant couple. As an example, these groups then begin to expand from childbirth preparation classes to family preparation encounters in which the couples share more than diapers. They begin to support each other as a community.

The atomic family offers a new beginning which integrates the individual and the collective simultaneously. The atomic family has the potential to be more inclusive than the families of the past. If nothing else, a personal need for survival demands that these communities transcend religious and racial prejudices. Such non-exclusive communities allow for a networking system that links up one community with another. But once again, can we honor our past by its completion? Can we resolve our unfinished business with the nuclear family before we evolve into the atomic family and thereby speed up our natural course of evolution?

The pre-existent family can offer a foundation for the expanding collective. Prospective grandparents can be an invaluable aid to their children. Grandparents can share with their children their own experiences and feelings during their pregnancies: an honest account of how this was for them, their joy, their pain, their doubts, their resolutions, and finally their recoveries. This can lead to the healing of open wounds that may still remain between the parents-to-be and their own parents.

Pregnancy offers a rebirth for three and often four generations. To see my mother welcome her first great-grandchild, Rachel, into the world and to watch her knit that newborn babe a sweater with hands gnarled by arthritis served to awaken within me and all her children and grandchildren the understanding of what the courageous beauty of age means.

It is extremely important during this pregnant interval for the expectant couple to reflect upon their own childhood in relationship to their parents. With this recall of the parent/child relationship, the information gained can serve as a model for parenthood. Now the pregnant couple can share their childhood experiences with each other and discover those behaviors and attitudes they wish to either emulate or avoid and those they wish to pass on to their children. Pregnancy is not associated with a biologic birth alone. It can be a period of psychological, emotional, and spiritual rebirth for past generations and generations to come.

The physician is another who is in a position to help guide the pregnant couple in those contracted periods of pregnancy. The pregnant interval labors and often demands an understanding physician who, through the experiences of others, can assuage the psychic contractions of false labor. If you have a physician who is not sensitive to those needs, or who coolly brushes you aside with "that's normal, dear," then it's time to find an "uncommon" physician.

The pregnant couple's anxieties are often related to thoughts about the delivery, the child's sex, or even to what his or her future adult vocation will be. We are inclined to live in the future. We rarely live in the now. We tend to think in linear and in futuristic terms and to live in fantasy rather than in the reality of the present. Our unrelentless striving is a part of the Western ethic that a man's reach should exceed his grasp. But what is lost in such a quest is the present appreciation of what is already within our reach. If we could grasp what is at hand, we would hold everything.

The author/philosopher, Ram Dass, wrote a book, *Be Here Now*. These words form a mantra, or focused thought, that is worth remembering and repeating during pregnancy, labor, and delivery. Such a way of being in the world allows us to be fully present at each moment and, as such, "be here now" is of value for us throughout the remainder of our pregnant lives.

The couples' fears and insecurities may extend into the second trimester, the next three months of pregnancy. This is a period in which some women may have a heightened desire for intercourse. This increase in sexual appetite is possibly due to having fewer physiological problems than occurred in the first three months. For the expectant mother, this second trimester may bring with it a feeling of well-being and a glowing sense of personal accomplishment. This sense of exhilaration overshadows the expected fatigue that comes from meeting the metabolic needs of the unfolding babe.

However, the husband, who has just adapted himself to the first three months, finds he must now readjust to the new emotional and physical changes of the second trimester. "If she's changing," he may ask himself, "why aren't I?" He has not quite realized or even acknowledged that he has. He's pregnant, but no one has told him. It is hoped that one of the partners will be able to recognize that the depression, irritability, isolation, suffering and/or anger that either of the mates is expressing is the shadow, the dark side of pregnancy that demands enlightenment, that craves to be delivered and freed. The feared shadow is a natural resource of untapped energy. When the darkness is entered it can transform the individual, the marriage, and the family. The shadow challenges the complacent, stagnant marriage to change. Don't avoid it. Fear will have its day, so face it on your terms and transform it to the light of understanding.

It is during those middle and last few months of pregnancy that the pregnant woman may ask her obstetrician, "If pregnancy is so glorious, why am I so frightened, uncertain, and unhappy?" The expectant couple may not understand that a relationship is not always strengthened by security. We can all learn that, at times, our greatest strength comes from the effort it takes to *correct* insecurity.

Usually by the fifth month of pregnancy, the husband is able to feel the movement of the unborn child for the first time. "My God," he exclaims, "I think she's pregnant." This realization often leads to a new set of fears. With that movement, he may for the first time in his life question his knowledge of female anatomy. "Where is it going?" "Am I hitting the kid in the head? Where is it—going?" Overnight, more thought goes into intercourse as he voraciously consumes any health and hygiene manuals he can get his hands on.

The husband may also experience various types of fantasies about his wife now that she is becoming the mother of his child. He may begin to picture her as the mother he knows best, his own. These "incestuous" thoughts might become so frightening that his ability to demonstrate tenderness, closeness, or caring becomes hampered. Confusion and frustration are often expressed and are temporarily relieved through avoidance. The need to hold on to what was, constancy and security, is more representative of our fear of death, of change, than it is an expression of our desire to partake in the inconsistencies and challenges of life.

I have recently seen a woman who expressed the same "incestuous" anxiety on having intercourse with her husband, following the birth of her child—"I felt like I was going to bed with my father—I felt so uncomfortable sleeping with him—he even smelled like my father." Are these incestual thoughts, or just renewed images of a child's love for a parent, that have been misinterpreted and judged by the now adult?

As his wife tends to be more secure and inseparate from the pregnancy, the husband, more likely than not, feels cast adrift and may even try to involve himself, both physiologically and psychologically, in the pregnancy. In such cases, the husband loses the balance between being an observer and a participant in the pregnancy. If he totally enters his wife's pregnant field, then he abdicates his own uniqueness in the relationship. This type of sympathetic reaction by the male to pregnancy often leads to a variable assortment of psychosomatic complaints.

Leidenberg, Trethowan, and Conlon write of expectant fathers who experience nausea, diarrhea, toothache, and headaches. Other husbands may tend to gain weight and even look pregnant. This is a sympathetic pregnancy. Others become so anxious during the middle months of pregnancy that they even become jealous of the wife's ability to perceive the child's movements. These men are inclined to experience the baby in the same manner as their mate, and may compete possessively for the child. These periods of fantasy can even extend throughout the entire nine-month gestation, labor, and delivery.

This is a shift in the husband's role of being compassionate, the state of being both an observer and a participant, to one of a sympathizer who becomes his observations. The state of compassion is a normal, healthy, interactive one, while that of sympathy serves no one. Pregnancy is a master teacher of this lesson of life.

Society also offers the pregnant couple a special kind of compassion in the second trimester. The wife enjoys reassurance from her friends, parents, her obstetrician, and even from strangers who spontaneously validate her state of being. Her external changes are easy to see and often elicit tender concern from bus drivers, headwaiters, or grocery-store clerks. Strangers greet her on the street and lovingly ask, "How far along are you?" Her new life's condition seems well supported and affords an opportunity for even the most reticent to make warm contact and offer uninhibited exchanges—"You're carrying beautifully." In a sense, she now becomes the universal recipient of goodwill. The pride she often feels is written across her chest and abdomen in the form of T-shirts that proclaim, "Yes, I am," or "Under construction," or perhaps there may be an arrow which simply points to "My baby." The husband, in the meantime, if unaware of his role, jealously quizzes himself: "What about me? What about me?"

The maternal awareness takes the form of a sudden desire to exercise and eat proper foods. Women who never were interested before in physical fitness now begin jogging programs. With this increased awareness of their bodily changes, some expectant mothers are even so foolish as to begin to diet. I cannot say enough about the importance of body fitness, but there is more to fitness than a slim body. To squeeze a Rolls-Royce mind into a Volkswagen body is an injustice. The body, like the mind, has its needs, its work, its rest, and its loves.

As the pregnancy continues, many women see their bodies as distorted. The mirror on the wall often becomes the enemy. The vain attempt to lose weight or to resolve anxiety may lead to bizarre, non-nutritive diets or the use of pills and other drugs such as alcohol and tranquilizers. These measures can be hazardous to the newborn and the soon-to-be born child who depends upon his mother's internal environment.

Severe growth and mental retardation in the newborn caused by alcohol and smoking abuse during pregnancy is well documented, as are the sequela of an inadequate protein intake. These are human-made catastrophies which are preventable. The laws of the body behave identically to the laws of the mind. The two are as inseparable as the couple and the child.

In the sixties, the New York Board of Education initiated Operation Head Start, a preschool program for the disadvantaged. The program was started four years too late. It should have started pre-conceptively or at least with conception by initiating an adequate diet and health program.

The ideal time to prepare physically for pregnancy is prior to conception. Any experienced bike enthusiast knows how difficult it is to shift gears while going up hill. The time to prepare onself for change is on level ground, prior to transition. This metaphor speaks to the couple contemplating a pregnancy in the near future or for those who now find themselves pregnant. Finally, childbirth preparation begins mentally, physically, and spiritually through understanding all that precedes, surrounds and follows one's own birth.

Society, too, has an obligation to protect its future generations. Nuclear power is an example. The potential of nuclear fallout and the inability to dispose of nuclear waste from energy reactors, for figuratively hundreds of years, is but one obvious example of society's short-sightedness. Genetic disorders that can be produced through nuclear radiation and then propagated through chromosome breakage are untreatable. The children conceived under such a cloud will be prophetic reminders of an unthinking generation that rolled dice with the future of humankind.

The rising incidence of certain cancers in children and young adults should be a sufficient warning to even the most diehard proponents of nuclear energy. Einstein, with the simplicity that marks wisdom, said, "Concern for man himself must always constitute the chief objective of all technological effort."

Finally, we come home to the last three months. The now very, very pregnant woman may experience still more fatigue. With the decrease in vaginal secretions, she enjoys intercourse less. Her shape has been distorted to its maximum. Rolling over in bed, tying her shoes, or sitting for long periods of time demand Herculean effort. She contends with the swollen feet, the swollen abdomen, and the characteristic duck waddle as the pelvis loosens for birth. She faces wild swings in appetite which range from sudden nausea at the mention of certain foods to an incredibly ravenous hunger at 2 a.m. She experiences more wakeful nights, more moments of exquisite fear and an ever-present exhaustion to match her erratic temperament.

The husband often becomes all thumbs and just doesn't know how to soften her doubts. Knowing whatever he says is suspect, he may enter a self-imposed vow of silence.

The couple relives the vaguely remembered horrors of their own birth—"My mother said I was at least eleven pounds—or was it eight? Sure hope our kid is smaller," or "I think I was the kid with the tight cord around my neck—I was so blue they thought I was dead—or was it my brother, Peter?"

There are also those repeated themes that are played over and over incessantly in the mind: "I hope I ate the right food—that article on cyclamates—don't know what to eat these days." Her husband, as if telepathic, responds in syncopation with her thoughts: "Did you take your vitamins today? You see that article on . . .?"

The above scenario is not always the case. In fact, it might be acted out as a self-fulfilled prophecy that was conjured up in the minds of early Hollywood. I know many couples who have continued on with their lives, uninterrupted by the many myths of pregnancy. Each of us is our own limitation. John Lilly said it so aptly, "What one believes to be true is true both experimentally and experientially. These beliefs are to be transcended."

The ability to resolve stress and to transcend insecurities is the hallmark, the *sine qua non,* of maturity—parenthood. It is in the ability to transcend and release moments of conflict through rapid problem solving that adulthood, with all its potential for creativity, is achieved. Those who suffer for prolonged periods of time with deep emotional stress accompanied by rare moments of recovery are stuck in adolescent despair.

Maturity is not measured by the ability to tolerate suffering so much as by the wisdom to shorten its duration. In the seasoned couple, the frequency of the highs and lows are not diminished so much as the amplitude of their rollercoaster ride from bliss to depression. The mature couple learns to suffer faster but gets on with the living sooner. In a sense, the seasoned couple goes through the fire of creative depression with less discomfort and more transformations. I now know what the Zen master meant when he said, "To suffer is to walk the first step along the path of life." In that knowing, *personal* suffering is transmuted to understanding.

Spinoza stated it simply and precisely when he said, "Suffering ceases to be suffering when one has a clear precise picture of it." The creative process is often dealt with in isolation. However, aloneness is all one-ness. It is knowing that you are a co-creator with the *Creator,* in creation. Don't run from fear, conflict or loneliness. The energy born of anxiety can be recycled in a positive manner. If all were bliss, creativity would be as vestigial as the human tail.

The essence of the creative process is found in the "big bang" theory of the earth's creation. Science tells us that through explosive, expansive energy, both annihilation and birth can occur simultaneously. Although nothing appears to happen within the silence of a vacuum, it is within such states that the omnipotent source of all creation is found. However, the initiation of the creation often demands agitation before it can fully be made manifest. As of this date in human consciousness, we have not evolved enough to serve voluntarily without stress-filled agitation. In the future the path of voluntary service will be revealed. This path is found through the joy of giving.

However, with our present consciousness, our uniqueness is achieved as a result of our choices, our risks, and our willingness to cope when agitated. When life presents events that test the wisdom of these choices, the results of our decisions will determine the quality of our lives, and our individuality. Therefore, it is the events, as well as the intervals that separate them, that determine the quality of our lives. So it could be said that the shortest distance between life and death is a wave that represents the composite of our risks taken and our choices made. Thus, our quality of life is so determined and, in a sense, the duration of life is inconsequential.

It is vital to bear in mind that the impact of pregnancy may be felt for years beyond the birth itself. In fact, unshared emotions between a couple can become habituated and thus programmed throughout the remaining years of marriage. These emotions, these negative and mistaken perceptions, have the power to cancel the initial intention of joy and can become a part of a life-long pattern. The converse is also true: the joy generated can infinitely sustain the already solid marriage.

For many couples, pregnancy is so natural and such a joy

that when the moment of truth approaches, birth, there is a reluctance to surrender their possession, their work, their creation. This moment of truth provides the next lesson of life that pregnancy teaches so well: the letting go of a creation in order that it, too, can survive. This is true of all creative endeavors, be they gourmet cooking, writing a book, or children.

I am reminded of a paragraph in Alexei Panshin's novel, *The Thurb Revolution:* "Near the end of any long-term project, there comes an inevitable moment when the end can be seen, but the hand cannot move. If the hand moves, the project will be over, and that is a monumentous thing to wish. Something inside suspects that anticipation may be better than memory, and wants to hold on to anticipation for a last moment." But the creator often fails to remember that the final completion of any creation only comes with its sharing. *Life is A Shared Creation* will be completed by your reading of it. For that, I will be eternally grateful. We are co-creators in this book.

If pregnancy is life, then pregnancy has humor. With humor and tolerance, it is easier to create in wholeness and unity. A little laughter goes a long way in making this a reality.

Pregnancy can provide us with some of the most memorable yet ridiculous experiences of life. Many of those moments are created by "that darn belly." It just seems to be everywhere except in front of you; that is, except when making love. Then it holds its own ground. If nothing else, "that darn belly" demonstrates how creative and resourceful a couple can really be. What about those untimely kicks which explicitly communicate the baby's preference: "Not again tonight—you're giving me a headache!" Or the "dry runs" by car to the hospital in search of the fastest route, or the mixture of panic and relief over being told, "You're in false labor . . . go home and sleep it off." "Why did I ever pick that turkey as an obstetrician?"

The Chinese have known for centuries that laughter, which is often referred to as "the cosmic voice of the gods," has a healing force. It is a communicator of health and happiness. Sometimes the spoken word just does not do it. Ashley Pitt has been quoted as saying, "The only trouble with words is that you can't communicate with them," so how about a hug, a kiss, or even a smile? They are all worth more than a thousand words. Books could be filled with information on what the individual or couple should do during pregnancy, but to be completely bogged down by "shoulds" and "musts" is to lose the joy of "the coming." It is to miss the mark of the pregnant moment.

Allow romance to evolve within your marriage. Romance is a shared creation. Familiarity has a nasty habit of dulling romance as each partner takes the other for granted. Societies' mass movements towards separation and divorce may be no more than an inherent drive to recapture lost or stultified romance. Our current quest for spiritual growth may be in a sense but another attempt to capture the lost formless aspect of love. The spiritual revolution offers the individual a never-ending mystical love affair, a love affair that is never consumated by orgasm, a love affair without end, a socially acceptable partner. To incorporate the mystical union into the worldly marriage has been the quest of humankind throughout ages.

How is this achieved? To live the unanswered question is the highest state of willingness that I know. Perhaps the question of how to have an evolving romance should be asked at an earlier age in order to have more time to live out that most rewarding answer. But it is also wise to remember that our new-found solutions are more often than not our next problems.

Time defines space and so encloses relationships. Both spirituality and human relationships can evolve by being timeless. Too often romance between individuals diminishes space. Love thrives when there is enough space to mirror oneself in the reflection of another. However, romance over time, intimacy, tends to label that dimension of space. Therefore, what once began as formless love evolves into the confines of husband, wife, father, mother, provider, bearer, or whatever. With these labels comes the assumed expectations, while the initial intent of formless love gets buried. Now the dimension of time creates explicit masks that define love as to its personal and societal myth of what should be. In fear of hurting another or being hurt, such a love soon evolves into unspoken dishonesty in order not to disrupt the myth of "shoulds" and "musts." Thus, love becomes distorted out of fear of loss of love. In time, these masks of behavior cover up the conditional grace of that initial, pure romantic love, but love's memory lingers on in search of love's rebirth.

Love cries out "Remember me" as it hauntingly seeks to be reclaimed. This is the same calling back to childhood innocence that once merged not only with people but with rocks, animals, dolls, toys and was so absorbed by life itself. However, to be stuck in that initial state of romance and innocence would also in a sense be but another type of death. Humankind's labor is to evolve both formless, unconditional and formed conditional love towards higher states of Absolute Love. The joy of humankind is to return once again to that state of childlike wonderment but this time with the wisdom and maturity that allows the arrows of "shoulds" and "musts" to penetrate, but not to scar. Thus, the joy of life is found in the play of life itself.

But even here and throughout the book in my attempt to explain love I have been adulterous. Love is pure. Love is wholeness. Love is space without time. Love encompasses all of life, all of existence, and so is free from definition, impervious to all attempts to limit it, label it, or possess it. There is but one love. To define that love is adulterous. When will we realize that our birth, our children's births and all births are LOVE made visible? Our labor, our work in life is to peel off the illusionary self-imposed masks and those masks of society that imprison us and return once again to the timeless space of the beginner's mind. Love evolves through the wisdom that comes with such uncluttered understanding. The timelessness of such a shared love demands the moment to moment innocence and honesty of a child. To live such a life is to live in a state of moment to moment monogomy, to be married to the moment, to make life the meditation.

The question is how can one live in the moment for one-self yet share that moment with another? Is this more California jargon? The answer is trust. Trust is found in the knowing that there is no separation between oneself and things. At present both the individual and society tend to be caught in a singular reality that is composed of forms that are separated by space, the physical world of structured reality. When something is missing or ajar in such a temporary world, we suffer a sense of loss, a void and so are catapulted into our most archaic and therefore our most familiar of all neurotic fears—abandonment. When we witness loss, we experience separation, isolation, and rejection. This is our heritage as told in the Biblical story of Adam and Eve who lost their secure place in the womb of The Garden of Eden. In such moments of abandonment, we lose faith in the less familiar, less tangible yet more permanent reality of interconnectedness. This formless world fills the spaces between structures and so transcends form itself. This world of interconnectedness knows no loss, no void, no death. However, the lack of trust in such a world of Ever-lasting Shared Creations is the source of our fear of abandonment, of flying. This fear has been the source of our contributions to life, contributions that have all too often been offered in payment to buy back our place in The Garden. As such, these gifts have been offered involuntarily, and usually begrudgingly. It is time to lose an old familiar neurosis. It was all a game. We never left The Garden. Eden is here and now. Abandonment was an illusion created by a race of children.

Humankind is beginning to understand the true meaning of abandonment. Adam and Eve are coming of age and so recognize that abandonment bears the gift of freedom. Freedom is not separation, nor hedonistic pleasure, but carries the greatest responsibility of all. That responsibility is to hold fast to oneself, to have the courage to be, to honor one's self as wholly human, yet to also honor the timeless interconnected space that integrates all things. Freedom is to live: I AM THAT I AM and to know that each one of us is living that moment for all humankind. This act of freedom is an act of responsibility. This is the responsibility to *voluntarily* serve without the need for prods, agitations, guilts or fears of rejection.

Marriage is more than compromise. Can you dare to risk all, even your marriage, to maintain the flow and rhythm of moment to moment monogamy? The answer to the paradox between self and others is to be married to the moment and to honor the contract of that moment with trust. Gibran said it well: "Pleasure is the freedom song but freedom is not pleasure."

No books, teachers, or parents can give you all the answers. Answers are those impossible-to-lose treasures which can only be found by you, within you. Answers are the gifts of understanding that you give to yourself, while wisdom is the living out of your understanding for not only yourself but for all humankind.

Pregnancy is not separate, apart, or even unique from other life processes. The pregnant interval is just a microcosm, a slice of life that obeys the natural laws of the universe. Therefore, think it through, act upon your thoughts, live with decisions, and bask in the faith that each morning brings the sun and each night holds the joy of that renewal.

Pregnancy is one of the many events that fills the space between our own life and death. Pregnancy is a lifetime within a *lifetime.* Like all other events with which pregnancy cohabits space, it is also a reflection of the whole of our existence. Pregnancy is equivalent to the chrysalis, the state between the caterpillar and the butterfly. The interval between conception and birth might appear to be a period of dormancy but, in reality, it is a period of dynamic growth, development, and balance for the pregnant couple as well as the yet unborn.

Yes, the unborn child labors throughout these months, as it unfolds through a series of developmental processes that reflect the history and birth of forever. In morphogenetics, this is referred to as ontogeny recapitulating phylogeny. (The development of an organism reflects the evolution of its past.) Whether this development reflects Darwinian evolution of variable species toward Homo sapiens or demonstrates that God is the interconnecting source of life in all things has been overly debated in both the past and the present by scientists and educators. But of greater import is that both theories share in the identical belief; that is, all life shares a singular origin.

In either case, all theorists agree that the yet unborn child is an example of the most extraordinary yet exquisite transformational process of life energy. The unborn is transformed from an undifferentiated, totally potential microscopic cell into a magnificent, highly specific, multidimensional form of energy. WOW! It boggles my mind. The full magnitude of this nine-month transformation still remains incomprehensible to me. Every babe that I have delivered has only increased my wonderment and my belief that there is something beyond me of which I am a part.

If the couple could occasionally focus their undivided attention and meditate upon that unfolding life form, then the nine-month period would provide ample time to transcend individual self-centeredness. Design your own meditation technique or bastardize someone else's by giving the meditation your uniqueness.

As the embryo unfolds and evolves through its total potentiality into its human form, it fuses with the two unique individuals in a Living Meditation. The unborn, too, gives birth—to parenthood. Where are the natural childbirth classes for the unborn? Can prospective parents be coaches for their child's nine months of labor? To be assured, the nine months are not easy for any of the three participants in transformation. Each must deal with his or her own uniqueness and so each has a specific lesson to be learned. But in the end, each shares in the common gift of life.

The joy gained from the fusion of this triad upon reaching the completion of their rite of passage can erase the most acute pain that occasionally accompanies the birth of any creation. Joy is synonymous with the birth of evolving life.

VI | *Inner sensory awareness gives birth to extra sensory perception.*

To Communicate With The Yet Unborn

Technology • Intuition • Telepathy
Inner Sensory Awareness

Throughout the sculpting, the sculptor, in quietness, touches the stone, caresses its surface, and speaks to it with love. He can smell the new surface, taste the joy of its completion, and hear its agonal cry to be born. There is a coming together, a loss of separation, as the sulptor merges with his creation. So, too, the pregnant couple can communicate with the yet unborn child. They can make the pregnancy more sensual and less distant. This prepares the husband and wife for their gradual shift into parenthood, into the extended family.

On one level, medical technology makes this communication possible. The baby often becomes more of a reality as it, too, communicates to all who wait to hear of its coming. To see the expression of a young child who may accompany her mother and father to the doctor's office as she hears her brother or sister for the first time is memorable. Her eyes all but leave her head as she listens in total disbelief, hopeful that the thump, thump, thump is really her baby brother or sister. This is not infrequently accompanied by soft tears of joy as the couple watch their child's expressions and share in the sounds of unborn music.

When appropriate, more sophisticated ultrasound machines are used to picture the baby and its source of nourishment, the placenta. This safe diagnostic test, which is called sonography, is performed to determine twin pregnancies, placental and fetal locations, or to determine certain abnormalities.

It is not uncommon for women over 35, or the couple who has a family history of genetic abnormalities, to have an amniocentesis. In this procedure, amniotic fluid is withdrawn from a painlessly placed needle in the abdomen and through the pregnant uterus. The cells obtained are then cultured (grown), and genetic and chemical determinations are made as to the baby's health.

If warranted, such procedures as sonography and amniocentesis can be used far beyond their diagnostic capabilities. The methods can be used to intensify the relationship of the three participants in the birthing process. As the parents-to-be hear their child's heartbeat or see the first pictures of their daughter or son defined by patterns of sound, or are informed of its sex and health, then that inner unfolding being takes on an added dimension of reality, a dimension which can be communicated with prior to birth.

In diagnosis and treatment, technology offers us gifts outside or beyond our own individual capabilities, while humanism points to the gifts that can be found within. As these two distinct, yet inseparable, forces integrate, the resultant creation is proportional to the relative contributions of each. An absolute as compared to a relative renaissance in medicine will be found in human history when *all* the aspects of the healing arts are included as being essential and incomparable.

Technology can be humanized; it thereby has the innate potential to further the humanism of its creators. This is equivalent to the child who reaches maturity, and now parents the parent. The same thought that creates technology can now allow the technological child to enhance the formless love that gave it birth.

Recent movies taken through the amniotic sac demonstrate embryonic awareness as early as 42 days post-fertilization. The unborn responds to light and sound and actually sucks its fingers. The child is aware. Many husbands and wives observe that the baby's movements even vary according to their own mood swings and can fluctuate with music in the room.

If indeed the highly emotional experiences of the day can be perceived by the unborn, then the pregnant couple can set a moment aside to communicate their quiet love to that most perceptive being. That moment would not be in vain.

The unborn, too, can be held in your thoughts as a mantra of love—the communion of silence. Meditation can be shared. Facing each other, with entwined hands softly placed on the pregnant abdomen, the couple can fill the space between them with a communal meditation. Hands are extensions of the heart and transmit the same healing energy of love. Now the Zen koan, thought puzzle, "What does one hand clapping sound like?" can be readily appreciated. During this shared time together, the pregnant couple will find that silence is thunderous—an expansive, all-inclusive harmonic of oneness that has the capacity to unify the three participants in pregnancy—mother, father, and child—into a singular harmonic chord of love.

To further enhance the prenatal awareness of the couple, I often suggest the making of their own personal loving tapes with music and words. When the mother-to-be has a moment of relaxation, she may gently place the tape deck speaker against her abdomen and communicate with that inner being through the closeness of familiar voices and soft music. Often, pregnant wives and husbands playing such a tape experience the unborn's response as repeated, perceptible, and predictable variations in movement.

Immediately following the delivery, these same parents, as well as myself, have witnessed that the babe's head and hand movements respond in concert to those same tapes. For these newborns, birth is coming home to a familiar planet, a planet of light and sound.

This has more recently been observed by behavioral researchers who have noticed perceptible movements by the unhatched chick in concert to its mother's clucking sounds. For that given chick, birth is not so much the leaving of a safe environment as it is the entering of a sound, familiar beginning. Should we humans offer our children less?

Whether listening to the fetal heart in the obstetrician's office or sharing in group meditation, or journal writing, the pregnant couple can become more aware that a living, functional being lies within the protective envelope of the mother's body. The baby is aware and that awareness precedes its birth! This should be honored and stimulated.

The sharing of pregnancy-related dreams is another method for the couple to bring the unborn child into clearer focus. Parents have told me that through their dreams, the labor, delivery, and even the sex and appearance of their child has been accurately revealed to them. These dreams are usually described as "more real than real—lifelike." Fear of rejection or ridicule by physicians and friends often prevents the communication of these most deeply moving and, at times, precognitive experiences. But nonjudgmental communication has a healing quality of its own which allows a couple to experience more fully the boundless mutual depths of their consciousness and their creation. A physician friend of mine, Gladys McGarey, uses the dreams of pregnant couples to assist her in the management of labor and delivery. She also has shared with me the prognosticating value of dreams in the management of her patients' medical problems.

Many pregnant couples have intuitive feelings concerning their unborn, a sense of the babe's presence, an uncanny awareness of its being which transcends the logical mind. This awareness is beyond either the expansive uterus or the intermittent movements of the unborn. This heightened awareness provides the ideal milieu for receiving a gift from your unborn child, the gift of intuition. Intuition is the key that unlocks the inner world of formless reality.

The difference between intuition and what can be referred to as our Inner Teacher lies in the degree of our faith and trust in the intuitive process. The more we have faith and trust in our intuition, the more likely we will be able to communicate with that inner source of life's wisdom. Extrasensory perception (E.S.P.) is born from inner sensory awareness. Intuition is inner sensory awareness (I.S.A.). This inner knowing is identified when we resonate, when we are harmonically identical with what we are observing.

The unborn and the pregnant couple already share in common ground and so as the couple focus their attention inwardly upon the unborn babe, they are more likely to share common experiences with that yet unknown child. In time, and with focused thought, as if in the meditative state, the unknown can be transformed and revealed.

The unborn and the newborn offer the parents an opportunity to tap the innate memories of their own past. They recall the moments when they as young preschool children spoke to their stuffed animals, heard voices in return, saw funny lights, flew over roof tops while their parents slept, swam in the fish bowls, hid beneath house plants, disappeared under blankets and played uninhibitedly with their five senses. Pregnancy reminds us of our lost innocence, the innocence that accepts all the wonders of life without understanding. Pregnancy can recall our joyous spontaneity which allowed us to be both a psychic fool and a leprechaun.

Pregnancy can be a time to give birth to our ability to communicate with others in our environment in deeper ways than we've known before. The physicist is aware that the apparent variations in form that are brought through to our awareness in vision, hearing, touch, taste, and smell are basically a singular source of energy which is transmuted into various frequency bands. Telepathic communication occurs when we develop the ability to modulate our frequency band to a shared one—to resonate. The common band of energy that resonates through all forms, be it mineral or human, atom or macrocosm, is entrained love. This is a love that inescapably draws us into the rhythm of life. Once you are swept up by such a love you know that life is a shared creation. Life is oneness.

Martin Muller describes resonance in his book, *Prelude to the New Man:* "The natural phenomena of resonance, which can be developed as a means of perception is basically founded on a deep love current. It is conscious empathy, involving adjustment to the wavelength of the observed subject." In a sense, when we resonate with another being, we become not only more than we are but we become one.

I am reminded of the biblical directive "For where two or three are gathered together in my name, there am I in the midst of them" (Matthew, 18:20). This phenomena happens where people in love, who come together in love, co-create the oneness that is Love. It is precisely this empathic state of love that I refer to as inner sensory awareness. This awareness is conceived in love.

When is such love experienced? Love is experienced in those moments when you lose yourself in another. It is a place of total mutual acceptance. In such moments of merging you are in resonance with another soul.

How do you know when you are in love? You know that you are in love by the responses of your being to the situation of the moment. Your being begins to harmonize with the being that shares its space.

How can love be brought into conscious control? Rather than love being a random process, your being can be consciously altered to harmonize with another person or even with things such as plants, animals, or minerals. Resonance is achieved through the conscious opening of the five senses in order that they can extend beyond self and merge uninterruptedly with life itself. You now consciously observe the variations of the patterns of your five senses as they touch "that other" soul and, in turn, reverberate within you. You become conscious of how "that other" life force affects your own physiology. Through such self observation, you experience the joy of *interconnectedness*. It is similar to the sonar device that transmits sound waves to the unborn's heart and feeds back the sounds, thump—thump—thump. As a human, you have the added capability to direct and then modulate the sensitivity of your beingness to whatever you consciously choose to merge with and so touch levels of knowing that transcend the logical mind. Words are inadequate to express this level of love. More common than not, tears are the only sign that this unfathomable wellspring of interconnectedness has been tapped. Throughout the rest of your life, although you may have periods of being lonely, there is an inner knowing that you will never be alone. The paradox is resolved when one realizes that it is primarily through loneliness that one enters interconnectedness.

And so as you integrate with life and your unborn child and unborn self, your mind observes within you the responses of your own sensate being as it is touched by that deeper love for the people or even the things that you are interacting and participating with. It is as if your mind assumed a neutral position, the impersonal observer state, that views, as if from afar, the two interacting participants (you and your observations) in that special moment of life. Thus, we can merge with the form and formless (the conditional and the unconditional) aspects of another being and so communicate with the inner soul of that person and even with life itself.

There are, then, three states of consciousness. There is, first, the "me" or the "I-it" observer state. Secondly, the "them-out-there" or "*thou*-I" participant state (what my environment is doing to me—not I-thou), and the third state of consciousness that observes both "me" and "them-out-there" nonjudgmentally, the impersonal state. This third state of consciousness is the point from which the parent, the healer, the friend, and the lover can compassionately observe the movement of the moment and thereby most effectively communicate with the content of that situation. It is a state that is governed by the rule of acceptance. The impersonal observer mind nonjudgmentally and passively synthesizes the interaction of life (telepathy) and then can actively direct the appropriate responses (psychokenesis). The third state of being resolves duality through unity.

It is not necessary to lose or even surrender the ego to achieve I.S.A. In fact, it would be a nonproductive sympathetic relationship. The ego is essential for compassionate communication and healing. However, when survival, egoic instincts are foremost in one's consciousness, "me consciousness," and then applied to human relationships, the ego ruler cuts off the impersonal observer state and so severs or damages relationships. It is only necessary to quiet or tone down the ego in order that the deeper quality of another being can be experienced. On the other hand, imbalance towards the egoless consciousness leads to a ship without an anchor.

The impersonal observer holds center-stage between ego and egoless, form and formless, conditional and unconditional. The third state of consciousness is like the mirror that feels the touch of the hand that presses against it, yet also is equally aware of another hand which is as perfect yet remains silent. The observer mind does not judge or compare which hand is the hand of reality or which is right or which is left.

The impersonal observer, like the mirror, simply accepts both hands. This state *can only be achieved in balance.*

The love that is found within the impersonal observer state is conceived in the friction of paradox and born out of its resolution. This love represents the epitome of balance and as such tends to have a short life span. This state is often referred to as enlightenment, and is what I fondly refer to as exquisite moments of balanced schizophrenia.

The impersonal observer mind repeatedly walks the high wires between conditional love and unconditional love. This is the fine line of acceptance, the still point, the thread of love. There can be moments of overwhelming fear and anxiety during such poised moments. However, once that delicate balance is experienced, it is so exhilarating, so addicting, that you are willing to risk a fall for the next experience. I have yet to meet anyone who is chronically enlightened. Hopefully, this is our destiny: to transform at the speed of light, to be poised between the formed and the formless life, the definable and the undefinable and finally between falsehood and truth.

I am reminded of the cancer person who spent an afternoon at my home and followed that day with a magnificent note. "Paul, as a chemist I always thought $2 + 2 = 4$ but my illness taught me that there is a formless quality of love that is equal to the quantity of my conditional life and so now, for me, $2 + 2 = 8$." Is it necessary to have severe illness to double your life experience?

I most emphatically believe that normal, healthy, well-balanced people experience auras, hear voices, or even feel another's emotions. At the same time, others can have a heightened sense of taste and smell that transcends ordinary usage. Some people might have one sensory channel which is more clearly developed or tuned in than another, but sensory systems are interchangeable. Therefore, what one might perceive as an aura, another human being may hear, feel, taste, or smell. For example, you can learn to feel colors or smell and taste sound.

I am reminded of Mike Pender's lyrics to *OM* on the Moody Blues album, *In Search of the Lost Chord:*

> Between the eyes
> and ears there lie
> The Sound of colour
> and the light of a sigh.

We are just beginning to explore the vastness of our beings.

Dr. Brugh Joy, in his book, *Joy's Way,* offers three directives for the experiencing of life's interchangeable mysteries. They are: "Make no comparisons, make no judgments, and delete your need to understand. . . ." The mysteries of life are resolved in the universal harmony of love and so increase the wave band of that love which now incorporates *all* into one.

Yes, I believe that normal, healthy, well-balanced people can experience other realities and also perceive the deeper emotional, physical, and spiritual qualities of another. This process of integration allows us to experience the phenomena of psychokenesis (the ability to influence objects by thought) and telepathy (the communication between minds without the normal five sensory channels).

Telepathy can be experienced during the passive, meditative state of "receiving" or being one, while psychokenesis occurs during the active, directive meditative state of "becoming" or "doing." In time and with understanding, it will be found that "to be" incorporates within it "to become." The need for psychokenesis or our need to create change will diminish. Change is inevitable. It is impatience that is the constant.

The telepathic sense is the sense of "oneness" that a

pregnant couple inescapably shares with the unborn. There is an experience of the babe being totally integrated, yet separate and apart. It is a paradox that is resolved in the vibration of resonating love. Pregnancy is a master teacher of life's hidden riddles.

It is up to the pregnant couple, as it is to any sensitive human being, whether or not he or she honor their own highly developed intuition. Recent history has shown us that the individual genius of such notables as Madame Curie, Carl Jung, Mahatma Gandhi, Helen Keller, Albert Schweitzer, Pierre Teilhard de Chardin, Martin Luther King, Sister Teresa, Buckminster Fuller, and Pope John, as well as the collective musical genius of such groups as the Beatles and the Moody Blues, stemmed from their willingness to act upon that Inner Voice, which is what led Albert Einstein to write, "Intuition is greater than knowledge." Intuition, the inner teacher, can be communicated through many forms of knowing, depending on the uniqueness of the individual or the group. Each person, even those within the group, by dropping a bucket into the inner well of knowing will tap only that stream of collective consciousness that is at the level of his or her own unique level of understanding. Even the collective consciousness has diversity within unity.

Telepathy (I.S.A.) can be creatively applied to communicate more fully with our family, friends, our unborn child, or for that matter, anyone or anything that exists or has existed within our environment. Energy cannot be created or destroyed. Since each of us is unique, it now becomes our responsibility to find our own unique channel or channels, to design our own computer system, and to perform our own read-out. At the same time, can we delete the *need* to be understood by others or our need to convince the more skeptical of our experiences?

During pregnancy, as in life, you can use telepathic communication most effectively for yourself. Be willing to speak to your unborn, and then close your eyes and experience your child's answer, but without the need to interpret the experience. What is her color form? What symbols come into view? Hear your child's sound—what is his tone? Feel his presence—where does she resonate within your being? Smell her essence and then taste the delicacy of his soul. Or simply ask yourself questions and then, objectively, unemotionally, experience the answers rather than needing to understand the answer.

Rainer Maria Rilke deals so well with questions and the need for answers in his book, *Letters to a Young Poet:* ". . . be patient toward all that is unresolved in your heart and try to love the *questions themselves* like locked rooms and like books that are written in a very foreign tongue. Do not now seek the answers, which cannot be given you because you would not be able to live them. And the point is to live everything. *Live* the questions now. Perhaps you will then gradually, without noticing it, live along some distant day into the answer. . . ."

Inner sensory awareness is a personal unique experience whose sharing does not require a similar method of perception but a commonality of being. Inner sensory awareness is taught through nonteaching. It comes from within and through living. In fact, even to attempt to describe this awareness in words is to falsify it. Words cannot describe states of nonverbal intuitive realms of consciousness, a consciousness or experience "beyond words," even beyond wonderment. This awareness may become so familiar that it develops a texture of reality that is almost palpable yet still eludes the confines of language or the structure to uniformly teach it. For me, the greatest gift of inner sensory awareness is to know, beyond a doubt, that there is more than me and that I am a part of that which is more than me.

The only difference between those who are referred to as "gifted" or psychic and other people is that the "gifted" are aware of their gifts while the others doubt theirs. Do you have enough faith and trust in yourself to speak to your unborn, to merge with life, to chance the unknown, to play the role of the fool? For it is the fool who is willing to risk the loss of acceptance by others who is most likely to find inner awareness within himself. This is the gift of loneliness. The

wise man's face is but the profile of the solitary, pious
fool's.

The most beautiful thing we can experience is the
mysterious. It is the source of all true art and
science. He to whom this emotion is a stranger, who
can no longer wonder and stand rapt in awe, is as
good as dead: his eyes are closed. . . . To know that
what is impenetrable to us really exists, manifesting
itself as the highest wisdom and the most radiant
beauty which our dull facilities can comprehend
only in the most primitive forms—this knowledge,
this feeling, is at the center of true religiousness. In
this sense, and in this sense only, I belong to the
ranks of the devoutly religious men.

—Albert Einstein, "What I Believe" (1930)

Pregnancy is a time for the couple to hone the tools of self
and marriage, yet also a time to explore and birth new realities. These new realities can be applied to expand the couple's consciousness and to create a personal myth that is filled with Love.

In learning to resonate with your child, you also learn to
resonate with all the children of the universe. The 1970's
were criticized by many as being the decade that hedonisti-
cally explored "the me consciousness." But in a very real
sense, this is one path to "the us consciousness," the community of humankind. Buber said it well: It is necessary "to
begin with oneself but not to end with oneself." Pregnancy
and its final state, delivery, points the way. The inner contracted wave of receiving gives birth to the outer, fluid state
of giving and sharing. An American medicine man, Ray
Eagle, taught me: "Humble yourself to receive in order that
you can more fully give."

Pregnancy is a period in life which teaches the harmony
that can be found in both giving and receiving and that
births love. Communion with oneself, one's partner, and the
yet unborn, nourishes each dividing cell of that unfolding
life and incorporates within the genetic code the spirit of
Love for all humanity. The child is the template of the
future and the tuning fork for generations to come—go play
and, more importantly, enjoy and love the folly.

VII

Birth is born in the climax of the symbolic dance between life and death.

The Birth

Hospitals • Physicians • Labor
Caesarian Sections • Delivery
Bonding

The sculpture is almost complete; the sculptor taps the chisel with slow, painstaking diligence. The agony of strained patience seems more tolerable as the ecstasy of the creation appears close at hand. In a similar manner, the final stages of labor and delivery begin with the intermittent but regular contractions which bring about the gradual descent of the baby into the birth canal. The cervix, or opening of the uterus, dilates to accommodate the creation to be shared. It is indeed a deliverance, a new birth, and a shared creation.

Birth and rebirth are like never-ending spirals. There is a continuous return to familiar places and events, but the perspective is always different. There is always something lost. Prior to, and during the entire pregnancy, the couple/child intertwine, merge in unconditional love, separate and reunite in the spiraling process of creation. Birth is born in the climax of the symbolic dance between life and death. Birth is renewal—the double helix—the symbol and essence of the genetic code and life's transference.

Since thought has its own life process, its own rebirths, it too suffers from repeated deaths in its longing for immortality. Conception and birth are the death of that anticipatory aspect of the eternal thought. However, the void is filled with new life to insure the continuation of the wish fulfilled. The pattern of uterine contractions and relaxation is symbolic of this ebb and flow. The contracted agonal state gives way to the open, fluid state and in so doing gives birth to birth in the moment of death—the wish fulfilled.

At the same time, the contractions forewarn the couple to prepare for the birth of their child. The typical scene includes the standard doubts: "Am I in labor? Shall we call the doctor? Is it false labor?" Then, the last minute scramble to prepare: "Should I shower? How long will it take to get to the hospital? Where are all those damned notes from the childbirth class? Do you have a stop watch . . . candy to suck on? Oh, wow! What else? Let's get out of here!"

Any differences which occurred during the previous nine months are dissolved as the couple moves in unison, as if magnetized, toward each other. While the husband opens the door with one hand, his wife may grab his other hand and self-consciously place it on her abdomen to both demonstrate and share her contractions. She prays that this is not a false alarm. The husband glances furtively at his wife's expression, hoping to see the signs of labor, and asks nervously, "When was the last one?" The drive to the hospital seems interminable. The husband is often torn between the desire to drive at breakneck speed or to cruise at a snail's pace so as not to jar the gift package. The husband, the provider, is now the protector. The final stage of pregnancy has arrived!

However, some women may choose to be without husbands, or may have husbands who are not available. They frantically call their standby friends, parents, or obstetrician. The surrogate husband does not have to be a male figure. The love and nurturing one female can give another is magnificent. Women have the societal freedom to express empathy and a type of communal, uninhibited love that is rarely shared between men other than in times of tragedy or war. There are also those women who manage perfectly by themselves.

It is assumed that by this time all the needed tools for delivery are familiar to the pregnant couple. The choice of the doctor, the hospital, and the method of delivery have been decided upon. Most of these decisions can be made prior to the last few months of pregnancy—either through hospital and physician interviews, childbirth preparation classes, or simply by asking friends about their own deliveries. Because pregnancy involves another's life, these decisions must be made thoughtfully. The more the couple share in the childbirth preparation, the more likely they will be able to orchestrate the delivery of their choice.

The proper atmosphere in the hospital and the ease of the relationship with the physician are essential to enhance the fluidity of birth. For many, the hospital has a connotation of illness and death, a promoter of fear, but it is also a restorer of health. The hospital is the first environment the child will experience after leaving the serene, protective surroundings of the womb. Generally speaking, the atmosphere in most delivery rooms is not conducive to warm, peaceful transition. The apparent lack of concern for the couple and their child is brought about by the undue restrictions carried out to guarantee sterility. But, in reality, it is impossible to have a sterile delivery through the birth canal.

Are alternative solutions to be found in home delivery? Many of the more humanistic approaches to medicine have come about because of the women's movement—more specifically, through the demands for change that women have placed on their obstetricians and gynecologists. However, these demands cannot be whitewashed by painting the sterile hospital walls with color, or even by placing windows in the labor room (although it wouldn't hurt). Not only woman, but all humankind seek understanding and compassion, with the full recognition that we are all involved in survival. But often in our zeal for the change, we miss the mark. It is often within the polarized state that we lose the wisdom and strength of our crusade. Home delivery is not the only answer. It is the symbol of a justifiable cry for change and a more humanistic approach to life.

The nurturing provided by family surroundings is essential for the welcomed birth—the celebration. However, a more secure approach would be to integrate the love, joy, and family surroundings into the hospital setting. To paraphrase Paul Goodman, we don't need new institutions, we need to make those we have better and more adaptable. But it is within the hospital that life support systems (although rarely needed) are more easily available. Statistical analyses of risk percentages do not apply to human life. The life you save is always 100 percent. It cannot be gambled. Both mother and child belong to humankind. The wise choice of the type of delivery is often dictated by the needs of the baby. The unborn also has rights that must be honored, among them, the right to be well born.

In an attempt to meet the request for a more personal, compassionate delivery, alternative birth centers are being built within hospitals. Some of the suites are luxurious and the entire birthing process takes place in one room. This allows the whole family to share uninterruptedly in both the labor and delivery and, at the same time, to enjoy a homey atmosphere.

The physician, like the hospital, should be previewed well in advance of the delivery. The selection of the doctor will probably depend on the number of mutually-shared beliefs held between you and your physician. Therapeutic success between the healer and the healed often depends as much upon rapport as it does upon the healer's technique. Other than the pregnant couple, your obstetrician (or nurse-midwife) is the most significant person in your delivery. If there is ambivalence or uncertainty, then both the pregnant couple and the physician should be honest enough to say, "This combination isn't working." During labor is *not* the time for lengthy discussions.

The search for an appropriate doctor can begin years before the delivery. During routine office visits, you can quiz your physician about his or her feelings concerning natural childbirth, methods of childbirth, anesthesia, husbands in the delivery room, breast feeding, and, for that matter, any other topics that come to mind. Physicians, especially in elective procedures such as birth, should be interviewed before contracted.

Often, the obstetrician's mothering instincts are awakened. Perhaps the reason many physicians choose the specialty of obstetrics is because they fit into the archetypal pattern of an individual who may be quick to respond parentally and officiously to others' needs. On the other hand, the physician is often unwittingly placed in this responsible position by patients who have abdicated their own responsibility. The future of medicine will depend upon the mutual sharing of both health and illness by physicians and patients.

Health, as life, demands balance. We, at times, need people other than ourselves. A healthy body cannot tolerate the battles of doctor/patient egos and pride. "Physician, heal thyself" does not necessarily mean that we must do it all by ourselves, but the statement does demand that we seek inner guidance. At times, that inner voice will lead to the correct choice of physician, hospital, medicine, herb, or prayer. In order to communicate with another—spouse, physician, friend, or child—or in order to heal ourselves or another, it is essential to merge with the formed and formless aspects of our beingness. The healer and consultant can be found both within and without.

After such soul searching, the choice of physician and hospital can afford you the needed confidence and tranquility to cope with those often harrowing admission procedures. However, in spite of all the inner work, you still may be ill prepared. It may begin as you are ushered directly into the examining room for the final verdict: "In labor, admit." Or, "False labor, home." The latter statement invariably makes you feel inadequate, stupid, and, worse, ignorant. It is hoped that the physician is more sensitive to the difficulty that you face in making that diagnosis of labor. Since the diagnosis of labor is made not only by the force and timing of the contractions but by the state of the uterine cervix, then to expect you to be 100 percent accurate in the staging of labor would be to expect all women to be contortionists!

If you are in labor, the admitting orders may vary, depending upon your physician. He or she may suggest walking around the hospital grounds until labor becomes more intense, or may put you at strict bed rest. In the early stages of labor, bed restrictions tend to have an imprisoning effect and can psychologically intensify the period of discomfort. In more "primitive" cultures, mothers deliver in a sitting or a squatting position, in contrast with our traditional horizontal posture. The choice of method for labor and delivery should be mutually satisfactory for you and your physician. It is for this reason that Dr. Irwin Chabon reintroduced the birthing chair to this culture. In a sitting or squatting position, the mother often tends to be more comfortable and can more effectively bear down to have her child.

Ideally, all these previous preparations and decisions will provide you, the pregnant couple, with a sense of oneness and openness. The moment of truth—the delivery—is the initiation into fatherhood and motherhood. It is through such a coming together in oneness that you are initiated through birth into the family. For either partner to stifle emotions at this time is to detract from the splendor of the shared moment. Yes, there may be moments of pain, and, yes, if the soon-to-be mother feels like screaming . . . she should scream! The transition into parenthood should be approached with humility, honesty, and finally with the acceptance of one's self.

I remember teaching childbirth classes and using the words "discomforting contractions" rather than "painful," so as not to program the mothers negatively. Following one of these sessions, I attended the labor of one of the students in that class and asked her how frequently she was experiencing discomfort. Red-faced, with fists clenched, she screamed, "Doctor, to you they may be discomforting, but to me, they're damned painful!"

So, if you feel like crying—cry. If you feel like praying—pray, or laugh, talk, or be silent. The moment is yours and you cannot be concerned about the impressions that you are making on the hospital staff. This is the time to rekindle all the facets of your being that make you, "you," and that make others want to share in your humanness.

Unfortunately, there is a special group, the doctors' wives and nurses and women physicians, who may preprogram themselves as to the proper conduct for labor and delivery.

They become so concerned about pleasing the hospital staff that they block all feelings—all emotions. The incidence of elevated blood pressure and emergency Caesarean sections performed on this select group far exceed the statistical chance. Could this be a result of their self-imposed restrictive programming?

Do prenatal classes alter pain tolerance by teaching relaxation and breathing techniques? Can the dress rehearsals in these sessions prepare the most timid of souls? Yes. They can create a sense of familiarity and confidence which can soften the fears that so often accompany delivery. But, unfortunately, some natural childbirth classes can inadvertently inculcate guilt and/or inadequacy if, at the time of delivery, even the smallest amount of narcotics are used. I remember one delivery in which the woman's first words to her newborn were said as an apology for having taken pain medication, rather than an expression of joy at the child's arrival. How can any of us think of ourselves as inadequate? The only time we are truly inadequate is when we don't appreciate ourselves adequately, when we compare ourselves to others.

For each of us, as parents or children, this experience of birth is unique and incomparable. Every woman who has gone through it is to be admired. I will never forget the words of my wife, Joyce, "After all is said and done, our three births were the greatest experiences of my life. Each was an experience that transcends words."

Just as the pregnant interval between conception and birth was of such great significance, so too is the interval between the contractions themselves. Relaxation and/or meditation exercises are invaluable at this time. To suggest that you can relax during a painful contraction is ludicrous. But you can rest between those contractions. In life, as in labor, the times to relax are those moments when you feel good and want to feel better. The average contraction lasts 30 to 45 seconds, and the interval between them extends from three to five minutes. So, during this pain-free state, if you close your eyes, rest, and have meditative thoughts, your perception of the oncoming contractions can be modified.

Most hospitals have a fetal monitor that displays both the infant's heartbeat and the mother's contractions. This information can be used creatively during the labor interval to further integrate the participants in birth. The baby's heart rate usually varies with the intensity of the contraction. As the contraction builds, the "readout" appears on the viewing screen of the monitor as a bell-shaped curve. The fetal heart rate in turn slows with the increase in the intensity of the contraction. The monitor can thus be used as a biofeedback machine to tell the couple when to begin deep breathing exercises and when to slow down and rest. So the sound of the baby's heart, as well as the slope of the uterine contraction, can be used to communicate a more effective breathing pattern for the couple. (However, if your husband has been taught to count down to the next contraction, similar to a NASA flight engineer—"You have three minutes until contraction . . . you have two minutes to contraction"— it is understandable why you just might "blast off.")

The intervals between contractions can be used more effectively as a period of reflective silence. Background music or dim lights in the room add to this special atmosphere. The key is not so much what to do during the uterine contractions, but, more importantly, what can be creatively accomplished during the relaxation phase. It is here that you both can focus on your personal accomplishments during the preceding nine months and on the work that you have already completed in the sculpting of your shared creation. This reflective, shared silence and introspective meditation allows you, the pregnant couple, to merge more completely with your soon-to-be-delivered child.

During the early phase of labor, a simple meditative technique for you is to close your eyes and focus your attention on the bridge of your nose. This can be made easier by placing a small piece of tape in that area. This meditation can be accompanied by slow, deep breathing, carrying each breath into those fingertips which gently encircle the shared creation. As labor continues and the intensity of the contractions increases, the deep, rhythmic breathing methods of either LaMaze or Reed can be reinstituted with this technique. Meditation is accompanied by a decrease in oxygen consumption and blood lactate and with an increase in the alpha wave rhythm of the brain. These factors are found typically in states of decreased anxiety and increased tranquility. It is not important that these physical and chemical parameters be interpreted as the cause of the tranquility as much as noted as indicators of relaxation. These chemical alterations that accompany meditation, such as in the increase in oxygen efficiency, are also advantageous to the unborn babe.

Acupuncture techniques, too, can decrease pain perception. Many of the acupuncture points for relief of uterine discomfort are located along the inner portion of the shin bone. The gentle stroking or massage (shiatsu) of these areas can be effective in modifying the intensity of the contractions. Rubbing the areas of the lower back with baby oil can also soothe the discomfort. In fact, any form of touch that conveys caring is always appreciated and definitely unifying. The brain usually can only tolerate but one major impulse at a time. This is referred to as competitive inhibition. Touch tends to be conducted to the brain at a faster rate than pain, and thereby the soft stroking carried out by a husband, coach, physician, or nurse is quite effective in modifying discomfort. Touch is not only reserved for birth or illness, but is essential for life.

In truth, there are no universal methods for this phase of birthing that will be satisfactory to all couples. To get bogged down in methodology is again to miss the experience— the coming. Birthing cannot be packaged or programmed. The labor and delivery room atmosphere should be orchestrated by the pregnant couple, with the physician or nurse-midwife as consultants. The ambience of the delivery suite should be left to the couple. Is it to be conducted in a traditional medical environment, or limited to the alternative birth center? For the most part, the child does it all for itself. The helping hands of the assistants serve mainly to guide its perfect unfolding.

Whether to deliver in darkness or into light or to place the baby in water or a bassinette is a matter for conjecture. The importance lies not so much in the particular techniques as in how the techniques enhance awareness, to alert all those concerned of the coming of the new creation. The pregnant couple, the hospital, the physician, or the nurse should be able to flow with the medical conditions of the moment. Freedom within structure can facilitate a birth that can be appreciated by all. A parental thought that carries worry or fear of not doing "the correct thing" may be the greatest deterrent to bonding. Any method that you will enjoy will be equally appreciated by the baby; the newborn senses fear as well as joy, just as two subatomic particles that have been separated in space are aware of each other's movements—*Bells Theorem.*

Many hospitals now permit fathers in the delivery room. Some even offer the father the option to perform the delivery of the child with the doctor in attendance. For a physician, this should be no more traumatic than assisting a medical student with his first case. To see my first delivery as a medical student would give the most inept father confidence, but fortunately I had a competent teacher at my side. (That delivery still remains the most important delivery of my life.) In either situation, both intern and father will probably be equally nervous and confused. But with the support of a calm physician, a clean, nontraumatic delivery can be carried off with aplomb. The long-term results of such a birth can be forever rewarding and may strengthen the ultimate bond between husband and wife, parent and child. It is the birth of both the child and the family into the collective bond of humanity. Just to think of it is overwhelming.

The importance of parent-child bonding has been brought to the attention of human behaviorists through the work of the Nobel laureates Konrad Lorenz, Kikolass Tinbergen, and K. Van Frisch, all animal behaviorists. These "animal watchers" observed that following birth, the siblings attach themselves to the first observable object that stimulates their senses—whether it be a moving object or a repetitive sound. These early learning phenomena are essential for survival and are imprinted or stored in long-term memory. The newborn animals become attached for an indefinite period of time to that first mothering object. If bonding is prevented by isolating a recently birthed animal, it is not uncommon for that animal to become permanently neurotic, and overly fearful of any situation perceived to present even the least threat to its existence and survival.

The question human behaviorists ask is whether bonding plays a similar role in human survival. As the unborn surrenders the security of its maternal environment to embrace humankind, it must undergo the ultimate moment of separation. After listening to literally hundreds of chronically ill patients, I have come to wonder whether bonding might not occur to other phenomena. Perhaps one can bond to emotions—for example, to isolation, rejection, or even pain, or to surroundings of either silence, joy, or chaos, or to sensations of touch or emptiness. I question whether isolation or rejection and a sense of abandonment might not be initiated with the cutting of the cord, only to be further imprinted by the physical distancing from both parents. But more importantly, the cutting of the cord is also life saving and freeing. Is bonding another term for the storage in memory of all of life's collective events? If this is true, parents should instill in their child at the earliest possible age that abandonment is an illusion and the only true bond is the bond of interconnectedness. The freedom that is found within interconnectedness is life saving and self-nourishing.

The parents, too, can sense this moment of separation and departure. This is felt even more deeply if the husband and wife are isolated by hospital rules at this time. Some degree of separation at birth is inevitable and probably essential. The memory of such an experience can allow all concerned to deal with similar circumstances of separation at a later date. The totally receptive mind of the newborn, as of the parents, imprints the engram of separation, and, at the same time, the memory of freedom that that separation allowed.

Could it be that the conflict between child and father, or

the karma of war and violence is due to either an incomplete bonding or an imbalance in the bonding process? Could this be related to the battered baby syndrome? Again, I don't know. But Ashley Montague writes in his book, *Touching,* that violence is often humankind's inappropriate attempt to touch and make contact. Perhaps it is time to extend ourselves in compassion for parents of battered babies and to try to understand more fully: What was their history? What was their childhood like? What have they been denied that we can offer? Can adults be battered as much through words, work, society, institutions, or even silence as by hands? Is there a "batterer" in each of us? If this can be recognized, we might be more compassionate. *Domestic violence is not limited to fists.*

If there is the possibility that the importance of bonding is a reality, then delivery again presents life's paradox—the paradox that arises in the very moment that the cord is clamped and cut—both bonding and separation take place simultaneously. However, if there is a delay in the bonding, the scales are tipped and separation can become more indelibly imprinted than bonding. Therefore, should it be necessary to have statistical proof of its good in order to permit this simple act of recognition to be consumated between parents and child in the delivery room and continued into the nursery? Perhaps even more so, the sick child that is whisked out of the delivery room needs the early imprinting of its five senses with its parents. Many couples have missed this opportunity and now at a later date, when viewing their ill child for the first time, question: "How do I know *it's* mine—are you sure?"

A mother came for counseling due to her concern over her eight-year-old daughter who had begun to show masochistic tendencies. She shared with me the circumstances of her daughter's premature birth and the breathing problems that ensued. For the next six weeks of that child's life, she remained in the confines of the intensive care nursery, restricted by ventilating machines and intravenouses. Here was a case when the needed life-saving measures, although painful, were, at the same time, nurturing. The parents, however, were not allowed equal time. I can't say it enough: It is all a question of balance.

It is possible, in those most receptive life-saving weeks, that the newborn infant bonded to pain, needle punctures, and restraints, for they, too, were offered with love and hope. It is also possible that what is familiar to any given human being in those formative hours of life can at a later date become natural and sought out either consciously or unconsciously. The seeking can take place in spite of what society may judge to be appropriate. Can this explain why an eight-year-old wants to play games in which she is tied down and tortured?

This case is similar to that of another child that I know who was born with breathing difficulties and spent the first three weeks of her life in the newborn intensive care unit, while her twin brother had an uneventful course and experienced rooming in with his mother. Now at four years of age she has repeated asthmatic attacks which are relieved more by the starting of an intravenous in the hospital emergency room than by the medicine in the bottle. These attacks are triggered by stress at home, occur at night when she has the undivided attention of her parents and relieved by the familiar support and even perhaps by the smell of a hospital.

It has become clear to me that the one aspect that traditional Western medicine had neglected in its quest for technological immortality is the biopsychosocial model of the patient. Technology's battle against death can destroy human dignity in the quest for survival. The fear of death often distracts us from our greater fear of life. Modern medicine tends to overlook the empirical fact that life is more than living.

Yet there is also a lesson to be learned from these life support machines and monitors. Can we learn to communicate as unfailingly, as unconditionally, to those children as the machines? These devices were designed by a collective human consciousness of hope and faith, machines that automatically adjust to life and death conditions and accept either outcome.

In times of stress, parental thoughts rather than being filled with doubts and fears, can perhaps communicate more of the objectivity and compassion of our technology. Since the newborn is born in a state of total receptivity, unconditional love, the child unifies itself with its entire environment. In this totally wakeful state the child responds to both spoken and unspoken words and thoughts. Can parents speak to their child and observe the babe's response by the variable change in either his or her monitored pulse rate, breathing rate, blood pressure or blood gases? It is not uncommon for infants in an intensive care nursery to reflect irregularities in their physiology in sympathy for another distressed child. This is called entrainment. Nurses and physicians may soften their approach to these children if they would begin to notice the monitors in response to their behavior and their handling of such newborns in the intensive care units.

Can we adults now learn from our own creations? Can we hold the vibration of the hope and the faith of our machines? Can we learn to accommodate more effectively to illness and death through the technology that we created? Can we also learn to accept the outcome as trustingly?

It cannot be said too often that the ultimate bonding process, the integration and unification of mother, father, and child, may take place when the father's hands are allowed to assist in the birth process and cradle the newborn. If hospitals and physicians provide the opportunity and the time in the delivery room for parents and child to fuse (physically, psychologically, emotionally, and spiritually) at birth, then the benefits of home delivery could be incorporated into all the accoutrements of the 20th-century medical technology.

Although a Caesarean operation necessitates a sterile environment, some hospitals are now allowing fathers in the operating room as an acknowledgment of their importance in this bonding process. These units also provide mirrors for mothers to enhance visual bonding. Dr. Cheek, during regression hypnosis, has documented the impact of both Caesarean and difficult labor and delivery on the newborn. Psychic trauma associated with Caesarean section was believed to be due more to the lack of communication between the doctor and the patient than from the effects of surgery itself. Even if the baby is whisked away, the parents must realize that they are forever bonded to that child and the child to the parents. Humankind will soon realize that we are all eternally bonded and can commune at will. It is our fears and guilt that weaken the bond, while our thoughts of love and acceptance strengthen this communication.

The number of Caesarean sections performed per number of deliveries has almost doubled in the past ten years. This is a result both of the increase in monitoring during labor and delivery, and the awareness obstetricians have concerning fetal distress and its aftermath. The public has been overly prejudiced concerning Caesarean section. Prolonged labor and delivery can be much more stressful and harmful than the surgery. To state that all children can and should be delivered vaginally is both an untruth and an injustice to those infants who are forced to share in the ego imbalance of their parents. Vaginal delivery is not always the most advantageous method for birth. Like consciousness, technology has also evolved over the years. Perhaps the obstetricians perform too many of these surgical procedures, but if there is a choice to be made between a difficult, prolonged labor or a Caesarean section after an intelligent, fetal-monitored trial of labor, then there is but one choice—Caesarean.

The newborn is a gift to the universe. The child is love made visible. Why are we so focused on how we unwrap the package? When we open the parcel and see the contents, that's the joy, that's the excitement, that's the celebration, that's the payoff. Why are Mother's Day and Father's Day on separate days? Surely it is more logical for all the participants to share in a singular celebration on the child's birthday.

In the words of Pierre Teilhard de Chardin, "Joy is the most infallible sign of the presence of God." In birth, joy infuses and then unites the creator with the creation. It is a moment of universal merging and emergence. This ecstasy can be shared with those who are close to us or who are compassionate in their understanding of this process. At times, the elation can be felt, heard, seen; it can even be tasted or perhaps smelled by those physically far removed, yet personally connected. The cry of the newborn, the most perfect of all human creations and sounds, heralds life.

For many, birth can be compared to the Ascension—the joining of mother, father, and child into the union of the trinity. Birth is deliverance for both the couple and the child. In obstetrics, the moment of full cervical dilation is called "crowning." There could not be a more fitting term. It is the coronation, the baptism, *a gift from Love* that heralds new beginnings for a king or queen. It is indeed a sacred moment and marks the end of the first stage of obstetrical labor—and life's labor.

The delivery is completed as the newborn unfolds like a flower from a contracted to an extended state and takes its first breath of freedom—deliverance. This is a moment to be cheered with the same emotions and sense of a collective experience the world felt when Neil Armstrong took his first step on the moon—a step for all humankind. The child is a voyager from space and deserves that same welcome.

Raymond Moody's book *Reflections of Life After Life* tells the story of various individuals who have been resuscitated following documented cardiac arrest. It is not uncommon for these people to describe a sense of joy and accomplishment as they float through a dark passageway towards brilliant light. This Western description of death is identical to those of religious mystics throughout the ages. The description also relates well to what the soon-to-be child may experience as it leaves the dark, yet secure nourishment of its environment to be reborn into a shared existence of light after the compressing pain of labor.

Are the experiences of fetal intrauterine existence metaphysically similar to the couple's as they journey through pregnancy? Carl Sagan, the eminent writer, scientist, and professor of astronomy at Cornell University, writes:

"Can it really be that every possible mode of origin and evolution of the universe corresponds to a human perinatal experience? Are we such limited creatures that we are unable to construct a cosmology that differs significantly from any one of the perinatal stages? Is our ability to know the universe hopelessly ensnared and enmired in the experiences of birth and infancy? Are we doomed to recapitulate our origins in a pretense of understanding the universe? Or might the emerging observational evidence gradually force us into an accommodation with an an understanding of that vast and awesome universe in which we float, lost and brave and questing?"

Each wave along life's continuum represents the composite of birth, death, and rebirth. Birth portends the labor and the rewards that are found within life. Birth is the stillpoint between death and life and, as such, holds within its moment an aspect of each. Birth is the "S" wave of the Taoist mandala that separates darkness and light. Birth is the pendulum of human existence that for but a flashing moment comes to a center point between the acme of its arcs and so erases relatively. Birth is the death of pregnancy, yet holds within that moment an entire memory of that life's existence. Every aspect of the birth process is a hologram of creation. But this is not surprising for every aspect, every facet of life, holds within its essence the knowledge for all of life. Life is the metaphor for life.

The rite of birth is no more than a momentous point in human time that is experienced and shared by all. It is as if life itself speaks once again: "Play it again—Travel on the spinning laser of life—Be willing to accept the path of love as well as the path of pain, each is your teacher—Have no fear—You can't help but learn—*That's why you're here!*" The babe cries: "But what am I here to learn?" Life softly replies: "To answer your own questions and to share your answers with me."

VIII | The void
produced by a
creation can
never be filled by
the creation
itself but to
surrender one's
creation is to be
filled.

The Cutting of The Cord
and
The Delivery of the Afterbirth

The Void • Engrossment • Surrender
Parenthood • Newborn Awareness
Knowledge • Understanding • Wisdom
Trust

The sculptor steps back and inspects his creation. There's a sense of disbelief in his eyes and he quizzically muses. Could this be mine? Could I have truly fulfilled this dream? Could these hands accomplish such an exquisite feat? Was there divine help? In either case, the sculptor becomes a pragmatist in transition or a mystic in total surrender. The creation is part of yet more than the creator. This type of enchantment and questioning mirrors the couple as they flow with each other and into the newborn. The final fusion of the trinity has been completed.

The sculptor also knows full well that the next work of art can only truly be initiated after completion and surrender of his last creation. The inspiration for creation must be delivered to the source from whence it came. The cutting of the cord and the delivery of the afterbirth, the placenta, is symbolic of the parents' need to let go of the child in order that they, the parents, as well as their shared creation, the child, can create freely anew. Thus, the energy for the never-ending spirit of life is regenerated and amplified.

For the couple to remain indefinitely in this high state of intoxicating birth would be impossible and unrealistic, if not selfish. Already, other aspects of life—other creations—

139

begun prior to this last but most significant accomplishment begin to tug at the couple. Family, friends, work, and even the marriage itself have developed their own needs—their own identities. These other creations plead, "What about us?" These previous obligations are persistent in their demands. The couple is often unaware of this process, and the two new parents wonder why their enchantment with the newborn has waned. They're apt to blame themselves or their partner. Those closest to us are often asked, and also have the capacity, to absorb our anxieties and our outrages. For some, if delivery is the icing on the cake, then the period following birth is the crumbs. It is difficult to avoid the depression that often accompanies the aftermath of creation. This period marks a new beginning for the end of a wish fulfilled. This is a variable time frame for the couple and the child.

The new interval along the wave of life begins and continues until it reaches the next momentous and universally-shared point in time—death. The rapidity by which we are willing to accept life defines human time. Human time is based on that unique soul's ability to remain in the present without attachment to the past or projections into the future. A lifetime is what we allot to ourselves. The interval between birth and death is not solely related to chronologic linear time nor can the quality of a given life be judged or compared to that of another. Each lifetime has the potential of being of infinite duration and, in a sense, life everlasting.

Therefore, to allow our initial thoughts and now our new creation, our children, to attain their full potential, it is essential to let go of the moment of birth and to give wings to our initial intention of love. The interval of life that follows birth is a further gestational period for the fruition of that thought.

Our constant interactions with our children cannot help but affect and further mold them. But the question is, can we interact with our children in the now without being tied to the past or the future? Heisenberg's physical principle of uncertainty states that the observer can affect that which is being observed. This principle could also be applied to parental attachment. Although involvement is essential for the act of creation, attachment must be surrendered to achieve the unfoldment of what has been created. This was implicitly stated following the completion of each new creation in the book of Genesis, "And so it was good." Letting go is a delicate point of judgment and varies from individual to individual. Nonattachment may resolve St. Augustine's dilemma concerning "the eternity of creative action with a dependency upon things creative." By letting go, we sacrifice personal dependency and gain impersonal unity.

It becomes clear that birth is not the end point in the drama of the act of creation nor is creation the end point of life. It is only one event, although a momentous one. The couple will never be the same; they have been changed through the act of creation—transformation. They may expect their relationship to return to pre-pregnant levels, but the nine months can wear down even the most optimistic of their expectations. In the interim, the creators have been changed by their own creation. They are not only a new form of the pre-existent husband and wife, but now a mother and father. This is a critical time for the marriage and now for the family.

With birth, there is the death of the conception and all its accompanying expectations. It is a time to reflect on projects and desires that were put aside during this nine-month period, projects that can now be renewed and enjoyed. This could range from enjoyment of a chocolate bar, to playing tennis or to returning to school. Pregnancy and the birth should not be looked on as a gain that was bought and paid for at a loss. "That kid" is often used as an excuse to refrain from doing all those things that you never really wanted to do in the first place, but which you can now rationalize into denying yourself "for the sake of the baby." (If I hadn't gotten pregnant, I could have been an astronaut." Or, "If you weren't pregnant, I'd be the astronaut.")

Now is the time to search out goals, both individually and as a couple. In a sense, delivery is the birth and death of a wish fulfilled. Post partum is the time for rebirth—nature's plan to ensure life's continuation and evolution. It is part of the infinite spiral of life. Even a diamond in the crystallization process of its fiery creation has unique facets that prevent it from ever again fitting into the void from which it was created. It is wishful thinking to anticipate that the void that is left after creation and after the end of nine months of expectation and now, finally, after the excitement of the birth can all be filled by this one child. The void of creation is never filled by the creation itself, nor should it be filled with resentment. The void is compensated for by the satisfaction of work well done and the exhilaration of a new beginning. A poet friend of mine, Richard Petitti, wrote in his book *The Sensitive Man*—". . . sometimes when you reach for a dream you have to leave something behind."

Physically, the mother is often aware of that void within herself. A physical part of her body has been separated. Yet there remains a sense of a phantom being within that craves form. Many women tell how they experience this uterine void—"A hollowness—filled with sensations of movement and nurturing."—"Doctor, are you sure you haven't left one behind?" This last question is asked frequently, half facetiously, and half wistfully, with a quality of wishfulness as well.

The desire to soften the pain of loss often leads to feelings of possessiveness or to the converse, the unwillingness to risk ever being that vulnerable or that consumed again. And so, following birth there is sometimes a period of mourning for what was, rather than a time of joy in what is. This may be expressed by an increased sensitivity and irritability as the maternal instincts to guard and protect the child are awakened. The mother frequently becomes defensive toward even the most well-meaning intentions of doctors, nurses, and her husband during this phase.

The guilt felt over this fear of loss and this inability to express it logically can become exquisitely painful. This situation can be clearly outlined for the mother, but knowing a problem exists doesn't always solve it. Resolution of conflict is achieved through personal insight followed by a personal effort to initiate change in one's condition—action. If it takes a certain amount of discomfort to produce overt emotional pain, then it is understandable that the sufferer needs an equal amount of understanding and compassion to resolve the process.

The multiplicity of physiological and psychological transitions in the family can lead to further bewilderment and anxiety. The inability to maintain an emotional high after this peak experience of birth often leads to self-flagellation. This can be further exacerbated by the added torment of not fulfilling society's image of the blissful new mother: "Will I ever get a full night's sleep again? . . . I hope I can at least finish this cup of coffee. . . . Can I go to the john? . . . Nobody ever told me it would be like this!" These thoughts lead to guilt, confusion—even fear.

The husband shares many of the same doubts and fears, and from the moment of birth may state in utter disbelief, "You really were pregnant! That's my kid? That's my kid!" His prenatal quest for "ourness" suddenly shifts to "mineness" following birth. For him, there's now a visible, palpable *raison d'etre.* This may lead to the phenomenon of "engrossment," a term coined by psychiatrist Martin Greenberg.

"By engrossment, there is a sense of absorption, preoccupation and interest in the infant," Greenberg writes. "The potential for engrossment in one's newborn is considered innate and it is believed that early contact with the infant releases this potential for involvement. Engrossment is expressed in touching, holding, and gazing at his infant and feeling that his child is unique and that he can pick him out of a crowd. Along with this, the father experiences a heightening of self-esteem and worth. The individual characteristics of the child—its movements, its alertness, open eyes, response to sound, and such normal reflex characteristics as the grasp reflex—all enhance the father's engrossment. His attachment to the newborn is powerful and appears to be something over which he has no control. This experience is even more acute for that father who felt himself to be neutral or uninvolved prior to delivery. There seems to be a total explosion on his consciousness, something for which he is totally unprepared—he, like his wife, now has a great deal of energy invested in the infant and the child becomes a focal point to rally around. The husband's engrossment following the delivery often mirrors the wife's autistic involvement before delivery.

Husband and wife may vie for the shared creation. The child can become like a wishbone over which each parent closes his or her eyes, makes a demand, and then tugs. And so the child, rather than the relationship, becomes the point of focus. The potential for this occurrence is enhanced by a holding-on, an "over-engrossment," by either the mother or the father, to the exclusion of the other spouse.

Is engrossment an attempt to gain a lost romance? Is the infant a new, yet socially acceptable romantic partner? Is this the genesis of some Freudian complexes or later the disillusionment between parent and child? Or can spiritual love be more appropriately incorporated into human institutions such as marriage and family? If possessive engrossment for one individual which is exclusive of others is a death knell to prolonged relationships, then is inclusive universal engrossment for all life a key to life everlasting?

Some parents can be overly dedicated and assume a subservient role. In this situation, the child's needs supersede—and even replace—their own. Or the couple may fear subsequent pregnancies: "How can we ever love another child this much?" They fear success as much as they fear failure. The husband and wife can either continue to be mesmerized by their creation, their irreplaceable possession, or they can acknowledge their miracle and keep on truckin'. To be able to relinquish the most cherished possession to its own domain of freedom is both a sacrifice and a gift. This is the most difficult task in the creative process of life.

But, in truth, to sacrifice means to bring an offering. To give, to free, to create, is not to lose—it is to give and then to free and, finally, to allow the new creation to create. Perhaps only when a couple adopts a child are they less bound by the physical and personal comparisons that often limit parent-child relationships. Although biological and emotional ties may promote intimacy and joy, these ties that bind us to our children, adopted or born through us, are more often subject to attachment. Attachment is the cause of the pain that often comes from separation as the child matures and leaves the nest. Through surrender—the phenomenon of letting go—we lose nothing, and more often, gain all. William Blake wrote:

"He who binds to himself a joy
doth the winged life destroy.
He who kisses the joy as it flies
lives in eternity's sunrise."

Too often, we, as parents, hide our emotions, such as grief or anger, from our children. We are overly protective and, all too frequently, present to our children a restrictive view of life and the transformational process that can rise above crisis. Parents fear abandonment from the child as much as the child fears rejection. Parents too often fear to show their faults, yet it may be wise to recall that the revered Jade of the Orient is the one that is willing to reveal its imperfections, its wholeness.

Paul Tillich in his book, *The Courage To Be,* said, "The courage to be is the ethical act in which man affirms his own being in spite of those elements of his existence which conflict with his essential self-affirmation."

Children can learn wholeness from conflict and loneliness as well as from love. Perhaps one of the most rewarding gifts we can offer our children is to teach them that disharmony can be a source of creative change. Children who never witness parental disharmony may find it difficult to deal with their own conflicts later. Movement from disharmony toward harmony brings enrichment and growth, while recurring unresolved conflict is destructive. To expect any couple to be in a constant state of either conditional or unconditional love is unrealistic. The problem lies in the fact that the closer the relationship, the more vulnerable the partners often become and, therefore, the more difficult it also becomes to sustain unconditional love. This tips the scales to the conditional level. Vulnerability makes risk taking more difficult. But risk taking is an essential part of the game of life. The more freedom a couple has, the stronger can become their bond. They bond to each other through their individual strengths rather than through their dependent weaknesses or the "shoulds" or "musts" of "the moral majority." The key to an evolving relationship is moment to moment honesty. This is a relationship that takes only one of the partners to say "no" but both to say "yes." In either case, "no" or "yes" is the commitment. It is the commitment to honor one's self and so to honor another. Like the Jade, to own one's wholeness, one's light and dark side, one's total humanness is to be truly revered.

However, disharmonious relationships continued solely for "the sake of the child" can produce children who feel responsible for the stagnation and unfulfillment in their parents' lives. To enhance the quality of our future, and our children's futures, it is imperative that we either set the intention to resolve a disharmonious relationship in love and thereby stay within it, or now dissolve that relationship and leave in love. In either case, we are no longer weighed down by our past unfinished business.

Love is the intention that can move conflict toward resolution and stress toward harmony. Resolution does not depend on anyone or anything other than oneself. Unconditional love can be sent without a return address; it does not depend on a response. This love is self-nourishing and does not need to be replenished outside oneself. Mother Earth, with all the life that surrounds her, is a model that so exquisitely exemplifies this love. She provides all the requirements for our existence and neither seeks nor asks for anything in return.

On the other hand, children can stifle parents. Some couples may resent the child for taking up so much of their time. The previously child-free couple must now adjust to a triangular relationship. This can overshadow the quality of the moment and, thus, the newborn can be viewed as a threat to the former dyadic relationship. Love is then quantified rather than qualified. Again, it is worth remembering that the new father and new mother should renew and evolve their precious relationship of lovers, and, at the same time, reclaim their own individuality. They are not only three in one, but also one in three.

People have their own unique needs and if the number of individuals in any given community increases, so do their divergent needs. We can see how simple differences of opinion, for example, about child feeding or about how one should respond to a baby's cry, can lead to friction far out of proportion to the situation. To breast feed or bottle feed must be decided by the individual uniqueness of a couple and their own needs. It should not be predicated on the latest fad or medical exposé. Like natural childbirth, child feeding is an individual decision and cannot be proffered as to its "correctness" or "rightness." The choice is yours and whatever the decision, it is perfect. Love and fondling, whether accompanied by a breast or a bottle, are the ingredients that have the nutritional wallop.

The sensation of touch that accompanies the holding and caressing of your child is often rewarded by the quieting of its cry. The child is not being spoiled, but the kinesthetic overload from touch may block the intensity and perception of its discomfort. The healing quality of touch is beyond our wildest dreams.

The model for this truth is found throughout nature. For example, ants incessantly touch one another in their daily activities and, in so doing, transmit a chemical substance which the entomologists refer to as the social enzyme, trophallaxis. An ant cannot survive if isolated and separated from this wondrous societal exchange. We have much to learn from all life's teachers.

Many children soon learn their cry is an effective form of communication to express the need to be touched, to be held. The crying infant's needs are not always met solely through oral gratification. In fact, this need to orally pacify may be the explanation for the two major causes of death in this country—obesity and smoking.

Fingertip massage of that most supple body and especially of the hands and back is another method either to pacify or communicate with your child. The thumb and hand have the greatest relative representation of the body in the motor-sensory area of the brain. The ability to touch the thumb to individual fingers (opposition) separates primates from other animals. The hand-thumb relationship plays an important role in prayer, meditation, the counting of rosary beads, or simply in stroking a worry stone. The webbed space between the thumb and index finger is also the major acupuncture site to relieve pain in the head and neck areas.

Does stimulation of thumb and index finger cause the release of self-producing tranquilizers? Is this why children fondle their favorite blanket or play incessantly with their hair? Simply put, I sense that thumb sucking is for thumb gratification as much as for oral gratification, and this instinctive need may be denied through the use of rubber and plastic pacifiers. Allow your child the luxury of its own natural skin, its own natural thumb. It is the thumb and hand that bridges the gap between the external world of formed reality and the formless internal world of the mind's reality. Hands are extensions of the heart.

I also wonder if even the mapping of the body within the cortex of the brain can be related to the random flailing hand motions of the unborn in its perfectly flexed state within the uterus. It seems that those areas that are most accessible to the groping fingertips of the unborn have greater representation within the brain than those, for example, like the back, which is barely recorded in the brain. This proportional representation remains as a constant through life.

Could this be a reason for the high incidence of psycho-somatic back problems in medicine? The back as compared to other parts of the body has the least familiarity and perhaps suffers from an identification crisis. It is my reason, at any rate, for recommending fingertip massages, especially of the baby's hands and back. The tactile system is one of the oldest and most basic sensory systems of the brain. It allows us to orientate the limits of our body to a spatial universe and to perceive pain as well as pleasure. Lack of a developed tactile system can lead to either a hyperawareness, irritability, or its polar opposite, numbness and apathy.

The holding and rocking of your child stimulates its vestibular or movement apparatus. This, along with muscle, tendon, or joint movement allows the child to sense its place in space. Therefore, the head and limbs can be moved through gentle ranges of motion to insure effective stimulation and development of these most receptive nerve centers.

The baby's cry should be thought of as a sound that does not necessarily have the connotation of pain, isolation, or hunger. It is a cry for all forms of stimulation. If adults can cry from joy, why can't a newborn babe? The child's cry is only a part of its language, a language we are only just beginning to understand, appreciate, and respond to.

The senses other than taste can be stimulated and used for communication. For example, the child's hearing awareness can be stimulated through music and intimate conversation. (A movie from Case Western Reserve University called *The Amazing Newborn* shows the baby moving in concert with the empathic loving voices of its parents.) The child's vision can be enhanced by varying the color and forms that surround it. The movie even demonstrates how the baby mimics the parents' facial gestures, such as even sticking out its tongue. Mirrors can further enhance this self-awareness, while smell can be stimulated through foods, body odors, and the perfumed oils used during massage.

Smell and taste are primitive senses more relied on for survival among the lower animals than by humans. (My cat's refusal of nonalcoholic Christmas eggnog after but a brief whiff made me question the wisdom of my own passion for the drink.) I believe if we allow children to smell, taste, and then spit out food, without slapping their hands or face and then forcing them to eat the rejected meal, there would be far fewer food allergies. Many children, in refusing a particular type of food, may well be expressing their innate survival instincts.

Our children are intelligent, clever beings who have the capability to communicate with all of life, even food. The society of consensus has embarrassed these innate gifts out of adulthood. These "little," "innocent," "helpless children" can guide us back to our lost past, a past that is essential for a liberated adulthood.

The newborn also intuitively senses our fears, loves, and joys. Dr. Edward A. Taub, a pediatrician, in a personal letter to me, writes: "Children often have colic because they swallow air. But often that is in families that are under stress; infants often swallow air in order to get colic. If parents react to this with fear and show signs of neurosis and worry, then their response to the illness becomes part of their children's experience of illness. This parental insecurity is often manifest in children as colic, school phobia, eneuresis, hyperactivity, wheezing, or constipation."

I also have a veterinarian friend, Bruce Cauble, who treats domestic animals only after interviewing the owners. He realized that the animals ills were more often than not symbolic reflections of the emotional problems of its owners.

Parents should comfort themselves with the knowledge that the infant reflects its environment on a moment to moment basis and therefore its desires do not always have to be met instantaneously. However, it should be kept in mind: whether sick or well, young or old, husband or wife, all need varied nourishment. This need may be an underlying reason for sibling jealousy. Parents of newborns often neglect the older children, feeling they will naturally understand the situation.

One woman shared with me her guilt over the resentment she had felt as a child for her sister, who was born with a "congenital defect." This woman felt guilty for wanting the same attention that her sister had received. As a teenager, she sought every possible means to be noticed, which included running away from home, drug abuse and pregnancy. Now as an adult, she has successfully fulfilled her childhood need and now gains attention and love through chronic illness.

Everyone needs care and affection. But when we are only rewarded in illness, then ill health can be both consciously and unconsciously sought. At times, it is necessary to heal the child-in-the-adult before the adult can become whole.

Not all our children are like newborn eagles—some can be dropped from the most precipitous perch at an early age to experience flight, but others, although they too have wings, need a nest beyond their twenties. Pregnancy begins before conception as a thought and continues beyond birth.

Too often, we see our own past or even our own creations as flawed. For an individual to refer to a child, or in fact to any human being, as "retarded" or "defective" in any shape or form is to rob that person of his or her inherent perfection. Our need to standardize individuals as to our image of correctness can produce children whose existence can be permanently darkened by the conditions we place on their lives. However, knowledge based on our illusion of differences that are born of comparison often becomes the source of our suffering. We can be too conditional.

Here it should be emphasized that phrases such as "congenital defect" and "mental retardation" are all misnomers. We are what we are, not what others want us to be. If we can accept a four-leaf clover, a mutant strain, a priceless rarity of life, as lucky, why do we judge a variant in our own image as defective, retarded, or worse—worthless. Implicit in unconditional love is total acceptance. Perhaps we are born with a certain genetic printout, but the quality of any life can be altered in the mutuality of love between parent, child, and all humankind. If the immaculate conception can be accepted as symbolic of the conceptus that is free of parental projections, then the immaculate birth is the birth of a child who is free from societal projections. How soon will our society be ready for such a birth? Twenty years? Two hundred years? Two thousand years? How many years?

As an obstetrician, I delivered a child, Lisa, who had a genetic variant referred to as mongolism. The parents were informed that their child would never grow beyond the mental capacity of a three-year-old. But Lisa's parents refused to accept the labels of "hopeless" and "helpless." Now Lisa, through specific patterning methods of movement, massage, swimming, and the use of language cards (recommended by the Institute for the Achievement of

Human Potential in Philadelphia), is able to read and can accomplish feats beyond her present chronological age. But, more importantly, her parents have continued, since her birth, to see her as beautiful—"perfect in her own way." Her parents often refer to her as a "gift of love—a gift without comparison."

Another close friend of mine, Karen Kenyon, sent me a copy of a poem that she wrote for her daughter, Johanna. At the time the following poem was written, Johanna was three months old, and her mother, Karen, had known since the day after her birth that she had the genetic disorder referred to as "mongolism." Karen wrote, "I have gone from complete nonacceptance and defiance to the beginnings of acceptance and love—to the point where there can be something good, something positive, a feeling for life in general."

For Johanna

Will you see the butterfly
  better because you won't
  wonder where he came from?

Will the flowers be brighter
  because you won't have to
  know their names?

Will you be able to trust
  completely in today because
  you will have no worries about
  tomorrow?

And will the world be a better place
  because of you?
Because you will not learn to hate,
  and you will not make war.
And you will not hold life to its promises,
  because it didn't give you any.

And you will be a part of everything,
  you will be the butterfly,
  you will be the flower,
And I will let you be all of this in me.

Three months after the poem was published in *Ladies Home Journal* in November, 1974, Johanna died. Karen once again offers us the gift of her poem, The Gift of Johanna.

I was personally involved in a difficult labor and delivery, the birth of Deepoo, an East Indian child born with cerebral palsy. Now, eleven years later, I have the privilege of working with this same child. Deepoo knows the cause for his spastic paralysis, yet he fully understands and accepts his condition. With an ever-present smile and with eyes that hold the wisdom of ages and the sparkle of eternity, Deepoo radiates unrestrained love. At present, his singular goal is to sit unaided. The love, joy, and acceptance he showers upon me has never been surpassed in my entire professional life. Who is the giver here? Who is the receiver? Who is the healer? And who is the healed? An understanding that encompasses compassion and acceptance can, through love, transmute the *apparent* differences found within humanity *from the suffering of comparison* to the grace of joy. It is not our problems that make life difficult, but rather our judgment of those problems. True, these children demand more work. However, they offer to parents, physicians, and all of society the gift of giving. But more importantly these children teach us the gift of receiving. For most of us and especially those who work in the healing arts, it is much easier to give than receive. They are indeed our master teachers.

So, too, it seems a possibility to me that Lisa and Deepoo, like all children, have been drawn to those parents who will provide the appropriate nurturing and stimulation for both their own and their parents' specific life work. The Jesuit poet, Gerard Manley Hopkins, wrote, "What I do is me. For that I came."

Our purpose for being here is a task not to be judged nor compared necessarily by our standards of good or bad, right or wrong. And this would all be equally true for both parents and child, whether in a biologic or an adoptive relationship. Or for that matter, it also applies to the single male who wants to adopt, or to the homosexual couple desirous of a child.

The developing child often completes the sculpture of itself in the image of its parents' intention and life's unforeseen events. To judge your child or berate yourself for his or her physical form ("What did I do wrong?" or "Why me?" or "If only . . ."), or the outcome of a delivery that might terminate in a premature infant, is to miss the mark. No one is at fault. Implicit in unconditional love is surrender. Surrender is the acceptance of the outcome of our contract with life without judgment, comparison, or even the need to understand.

Even in the most harmonious births and childhoods, the child can choose to misinterpret its surroundings and pattern its life around those misinterpretations. It is no more fitting for parents to accept the entire blame and guilt for their children's problems than to take all the laurels for their successes. Much of the guilt a parent feels over a child's unhappiness is totally unwarranted. In one sense, happiness is an autistic gift, a gift that we can only give to ourselves. It is also the responsibility of the child to transform parental thoughts and knowledge into personal realities and understanding.

As the moon is the lesser light and a reflection of the sun, so is knowledge the lesser light of wisdom. In a similar manner, even the fullest of all moons or the greatest of all knowledge is also half in the dark. However, in the willingness to allow our children to go through the dark side of their moon, we allow them the freedom to find wisdom for themselves. Knowledge is not to be dismissed. Knowledge is a gift the parents give their children and is the fabric of communication, while understanding is a gift the children give to themselves. Wisdom, on the other hand, is understanding lived over time.

Since knowledge is based on comparison, it offers us choices in life and allows us to express free will. It is precisely the choices we make that are responsible for either our suffering or our joy. Knowledge is the father of paradoxes and the mother of understanding. We know that love is the source of all things and paradoxes are but games that teach the balance that is found in all things. Yet, in spite of this understanding, the child must be exposed to the lesser love of knowledge, the fires of comparison, in order to be tempered by the greater love of wisdom. Wisdom is the understanding, gained through time and experience, that leads us to accept love as the common denominator in all things.

The parent's role is to offer the child knowledge, knowing full well that the child's choices can lead to suffering. However, the wise parent also knows that humankind's suffering stems more from the personal and external judgments of our life decisions than from the choices themselves. Even the most disharmonious decisions can lead to future understanding and therefore to growth. So the parents must often bear in patience the anguish of silence as their child is allowed the luxury of misunderstanding, the gift of suffering.

It is during this phase, symbolically represented by the afterbirth, that the parent assumes the role of a loving, yet temporary, teacher. Since the afterbirth period begins with the child's birth and extends to the child's independence, this interval of time demands even more patience and understanding from parents than the pregnant interval itself.

Over the years, the great teachers have always taken the gold of their understanding and converted it back to elemental knowledge in order to communicate more fully with their students. There is always the risk that the scholars might distort truth in their sharing. This risk is compensated for by the teachers' hope that their students, in time, will transmute their learned knowledge into greater wisdom, even greater than their masters.

D. T. Suzuki, the famous Zen master, wrote, "If the author is worth anything, be sure you will not get at his meaning all at once—nay, that at his whole meaning you will not for a long time arrive in anywise. Not that he does not say what he means, and in strong words, too. But in a hidden way and in parable, in order that he may be sure you want it." This could have just as well have been written for parents.

To strive toward "perfect" communication yet to accept the misinterpretation of imperfect communication is not only the risk of scholars and scientists, but a hallmark of a mature nurturing parent.

The knowledge we communicate as parents will never be totally representative of our understanding. It is a paradox, for although our understanding may be clear, true, and pure, when it is shared as knowledge through the conventional forms of communication, our understanding is more often than not distorted. Therefore, knowledge is the vehicle for both future understanding as well as misunderstanding, but in either case, an effective learning vehicle. Knowledge is a painful, magnificent, joyous paradox that often keeps us and our children in a highly pitched state of anxiety.

The parent suggests to the infant that there are choices on earth. There is the tree of everlasting life—interconnectedness—and there is the tree of knowledge—separation. With knowledge that has no understanding, the child often creates a false parent, a parent separate and apart from itself. The wise parent, however, bears the ignorance and, at times, wrathfulness of the child. The wise parent *understands* that knowledge based on comparison is an illusion. Comparison leads to separation and separation, too, is a child's illusion, blind to the source and binding power found within all creations—love.

No matter how great our newly found wisdom, when it is dissected and revealed to our children, it will never express our true understanding. This is what the generation gap is— the blind spot—the result of frustration born from the loss of understanding between the parent and the child. It does not mean that language is hopeless or does not serve a significant purpose but that it may be time for humankind to seek a more universal method of communication.

Inner sensory awareness (I.S.A.) is that universal method of communication that has the force to transcend time and space. This inviolate love is the energy that is channeled through the shared spiritual bonds that link one soul to another for eternity. It is not a love that directs, but an absolute love that can even accept nonacceptance. While the child goes through the pain of "doing" to appease a parent, or the adolescent stage of "becoming" to prove itself to itself, the parent holds the vibration of "being," the state of acceptance, even if that means on occasion, opposition.

Parental love is a presence which is more often acknowledged in silence or a whispered "oh" that accompanies total self-awareness. In truth, there is but one love and that love cannot be qualified or quantified, but only lived. That inner love is the part of you that is found in all things. It is the part of the collective unconsciousness of all existence and more. Love is the undefinable resonating energy of life.

In the *formless* state, love is that essence that pervades and envelops all creation and is often referred to as energy, spirit, God or all. Truly, this energy is reflected in each individual as his or her own soul, Inner Teacher, or self. Love is the same frequency band that unites mother, father, and child. But confusion arises when unconditional love is brought into concrete form or that reality in which formless energy is converted into the slower vibration characteristic of matter.

In the formed state, our senses label the conditions of love in accordance with its relative size, shape, color, etc. This type of learning is based on knowledge (comparison) rather than on understanding which accepts the similarities and dissimilarities in all things. Both aspects of knowing the formless and the form are essential and incomparable, and provide the foundation for wisdom. The question is, can we be apart and a part simultaneously?

The afterbirth is therefore a variable time frame during which the parents truly labor to give freedom of knowledge to their child and also attempt to gain wisdom and freedom for themselves. If the parents demand that their child leave in order to become a more active participant in life, then participation would be forced, involuntary, and would reflect more the parents' needs than the child's. Although tension may be a prime mover for growth and creativity, the *demand* or *need* to create change can abort its fruition. Creation comes with time and from within. However, an occasional prod or encouragement to take wing would not hurt.

Each phase of pregnancy labors. Parents would benefit more by orchestrating rather than directing the lives of their children. At times, this calls for the sharing of knowledge while, at other times, for the dispensing of discipline. Discipline is the balance between mercy and justice.

Even misunderstood discipline can spark self-awareness and direct childhood fantasy and bliss toward adult creativity. Although this can lead the child to feelings of rejection and loneliness, it more often than not leads to self-discovery, and with self-discovery, a renewed sense, a renewed awareness, a renewed understanding of him or herself and, in turn, of all humanity. "Discipline" and "disciple" share the same root word, "discipul," which means to follow in love.

The discipline of "don't do" can be an effective prime mover of doing. A properly orchestrated parental negative intention is an irresistible temptation that often directs the child toward the path of self-discovery.

The most beautifully orchestrated negative intent of all creation is found in the book of Genesis, "But of the tree of knowledge of good and evil, thou shall not eat of it." This statement has had the power to drive humankind relentlessly through the ages to learn, to create, and to serve in their attempt to regain Eden. However, through such a negative directive and through fear of a wrathful reprisal for disobedience, Eden has prospered—as was God's infinitely wise intention—an intention directed to infants. But have we come of age? Can we make voluntary contributions to Eden, to Earth through the joy of giving, rather than through the fear of abandonment or the guilt of noncompliance? Such involuntary service is adolescent.

The path of service is similar to the path of the hero that the anthropologist and mythologist, Joseph Campbell, refers to. The three phases the hero must go through are separation, instruction, and return. So, too, the child through discipline learns knowledge and through separation learns understanding (adolescence); then in time, he returns home as a young adult to share the laurels of wisdom: that sin, separation and comparison are illusion created through the misunderstanding of life's love.

The child thus matures into the wise teacher who now serves and makes offerings voluntarily. Our gift to life is that part of ourselves that is found during self-discovery which craves to be shared with another. It is often those conditions imposed through discipline that lead to voluntary service. Whether one ascends Jacob's ladder for understanding or now descends the ladder for inner wisdom, for movement to occur, it becomes essential for both parent and child to relinquish their perch each step of the way. The pregnant interval called the afterbirth demands balance, patience, discipline, surrender, and finally, trust.

It becomes clear that our creations are finalized not by birth alone, but in their own maturation and sharing. Thus, our children became co-creators in creation and thereby share with us and all humankind in the wondrous evolution of life. Meanwhile, the parents must wait in patience for their child to gain this wisdom. In the pregnant moment of their child's enlightenment, childbirth is completed for the parents as they bite their tongues to avoid shouting, "I told you so!—It's about time!"

This protracted and variable waiting period before the parents finally shed their placenta offers the pregnant couple another chance to touch but once again the child within. The afterbirth is a time to re-explore those same relationships with their own parents. All too often, our children's difficulties in life were, and still are, ours, and far too often, we respond as our parents responded to us. The afterbirth offers us a chance to use the farsightedness that comes with age to complete objectivity, or at least clarify, our past, and thereby revitalize our present. We can now honor our children as reawakeners of the child and the parent within us all. *When was your innocence lost?*

Maybe the drive that motivates us to bear children is our

longing to rekindle that lost innocence or incompleteness of our own childhood and to allow us a second chance to create ourselves anew. But, more importantly, this rebirth can provide us with more acceptance for our children, our parents, and others.

Perhaps, in time, some of our children will repeat the life cycle as fresh unique individuals who will merge to share in creation, pregnancy, and so in life. Can they avoid coloring their thoughts and shared gifts with our history, or dreams, and our aspirations? This is perhaps one of their greatest challenges.

Symbolically and prophetically the twenty-second chapter of Genesis depicts the end stage of parenthood. Here, Abraham offers his most cherished possession, Isaac, as a sacrifice, a gift to the creator, and so Abraham becomes the father of all nations. The final stage of parenthood is reached when the parents surrender that most beloved possession, their child, to the universe. The surrendering of our most beloved creation is offered as a token of our trust in life, for life. In that final act of trust, faith beyond understanding, the parents complete the gestational period of their own lives and in that wholeness, solve the paradox of separation. They are now ready for the next epoch. In that final moment, the child is free to begin the same riddle of life that has been completed by its parents.

The life that is conceived in the formless thought gives birth to the formed embryo and its nourishment, the placenta. The cutting of the cord that bonds the child to the afterbirth heralds the birth of the babe. In obstetrics this act finalizes the second stage of labor and is symbolic of the second stage of that child's life, the first being in utero. It is prophetic that this first symbolic breath of life should be one of inspiration. This gesture completes the transformation of formless life energy into form. The cycle that began with the inspirational thought of unconditional love is now completed upon the expiration of conditional life.

And so we see that in the moment of separation between the creator and those things created, the child learns the knowledge of breath. Breath is life and life is both work and joy. Repeated episodes of separation and loneliness in the future will often lead the child to further self-discovery, understanding, and service—adulthood. What appears to begin as separation is the initiator of the coming home process.

The third and last stage of labor is marked by the act of placental shedding, appropriately called the delivery of the afterbirth. This final gesture is a metaphor for the type of parental nourishment that is needed beyond the delivery and also, the metaphor to teach what is necessary for the rebirth of creatorhood. The cord has been cut and so that nourishment must come again through the formless thought of love. The creators of that initial thought are now free to create anew. To deliver is to give an offering, a gift, a sacrifice. To deliver is to free oneself in order to begin but once again the act of creation.

Detachment, surrender, does not mean a withdrawal of parental support, but a trust in life. Love's eternal labor, its wave of contraction and relaxation, co-creation and surrender, is what interconnects us with our children, our children's children, and the rest of humanity—not our possessiveness. There is never a loss, never a separation, but only an aspiring continuum to fill life's apparent void.

Full maturity is only reached in that final, yet necessary, stage of trust. In that moment, the ageless process of parenthood is passed to the next generation. The mature adult's life, as the child's, does not end here. The wisdom that is attained through the various stages of life serves the "grand" parent and supports all the children of the universe and all creations. The "grand" parent can hold the vibration of love. There is loss of discernment, loss of possessiveness, and what remains is acceptance. There is no longer a need to do or a need to become, but only a natural desire to be. The parent has gained wisdom, wholeness, and a long-awaited rest—and so deserves the title "grand."

The ascending spirit of life and its eternal continuum can be clearly viewed through the transparency of birth. Birth is but only one of many metaphors for love's perpetuation and evolution of itself. The life process that began in thought has no end.

IX

Love, like life, is pregnant and, as the thousand-petaled lotus, continues to unfold.

The Beginning

Love

Soon humankind will accept what the physicists of today are currently documenting and what the sages of old knew. Life is energy. And human life, like energy, cannot be created or destroyed; each form, although unique, is transformed from the same source of energy. Neither the quality nor quantity of human life, be it an abortion, a stillborn, or an adult, can be judged by our concept of time, good or bad, right or wrong. Death, like life, is part of this same illusion. Humankind is no more than recycled energy in transitional states of becoming less and less dense and evolving towards the more diaphanous state of light. A human's lifetime will be marked by the time spent on the wave of the now, rather than calculated by the chronologic linear void between life and death. With such self-realization of time, both the quality and quantity of existence will be in the hands of the individual.

If matter is no more than a form of energy in slow motion and death is the stillpoint state of that energy, then perhaps we can view our present existence (the one we call life) as the closest we ever come to death. In the evolution of consciousness, we are achieving states of less density, and our lives, whether viewed through the various psychotherapies, news broadcasts, or television "soaps," have made human life more transparent, more human than human. Yet with each new moment of self-realization, we enter further into a deeper understanding of the larger collective consciousness which pervades all creations of the universe. Life is a never-ending spiral of self-realization which feeds this evolving collective. Perhaps the ultimate reason for being is to learn to accept our humanness. I feel that this is both the cosmic joke and the cosmic prayer.

For me, the second law of thermodynamics—entropy—will be understood to be more than the disintegration of a system towards randomness. Entropy is also the initial step in renewal and in the return to the source of all things—ABSOLUTE LOVE. Therefore, change and impermanence will no longer be feared or avoided but will be honored and appreciated as part of the continuum of life's creative spirit. This insight will lead us to create voluntarily and to share joyously our most cherished possessions.

If this view of energy is accepted, the next logical progression would be to assume that there must be preconceptive life energy—the child to be conceived—and that that life energy is a co-creator with the parental energy in its own making. Thus, two energies fuse to create a third energy whose essence is still one with all energy. The preconceptive formless energy field and the parental formless thought field are drawn to each other as if magnetized. This union is *The Gift of Love.* The bond between these fields is finally consummated in the spark of physical love. In the dance between energy and matter, force and resistance, giving and receiving, male and female, a new creation emerges, synthesized from the multiple still-points of contact between disparate forms of a singular source of energy. Finally, the formed genetic code and the formless psychic states of energy are transformed into a new human being. The transformational dance of life leads to *The Gift to Life.* In that moment of birth, love is made visible.

This magnetic selection and union that is both the genesis and matrix of the family is just as true for single, adoptive, or step-parents. There is order in the universe, and all parents are temporary surrogates for all children. Parents and children share the roles of teacher and student, each learning from the other. Life is a co-creative process. When the lessons of life are missed, then a new generation is faced with the same old, unfinished business. It is disheartening to see a great-grandchild living the identical experiences of its great-grandparent. This situation, however, also holds a wonderment, a wonderment that is found in the order in all things and the eternal patience and love of life for life.

Once the union of the three participants of pregnancy has been consummated, the *quality* of each of their individual lives will depend upon the degree to which each member is willing to accept the responsibility for his or her personal contract with life. Therefore, it is not only the thought that shapes form, but the agreed-upon conditions that envelop the formative creation. The responses of the mother, father, and child to those contracts can either embellish or shatter the shared work of art. The ideal role of the parent is then one of a protective, loving orchestrator who views all of his or her children without comparison but offers a balance of conditional and unconditional love. This intention of love can serve as the foundation upon which all three can now build their own gifts to life.

> Your children are not your children.
> They are the sons and daughters of Life's
> longing for itself.
> They come through you but not from you
> And though they are with you yet they
> belong not to you.
> Kahlil Gibran,
> *The Prophet*

Therefore, the husband, the wife, the father, the mother, and the child will continue to touch, to part, and to reunite in interlocking spirals. They will draw their own conclusions based on their unique perceptions of similar experiences. To demand unfailing commonality of experiences, or even hold on to what was or should be, is only to temporarily divert the flow and rhythm of life. Although to resonate is to communicate, prolonged uninterrupted resonating systems can be too harsh, too shattering, even too abrasive for creative transformation. Again, balance is needed.

The perceptions of parents and children are (thank God) not the same. There is, however, unity in diversity, for in self-discovery, you learn that there is no separation from all that you have met, nor can the totality of all existence continue without your unique presence. The pain of separation can be relinquished through the acceptance of interconnectedness and so bathed in the grace of unity.

The fusion in joy and the parting in acceptance is the dance of love, and in this dance, all the parents and children of the universe rise again and again as individuals. Like the Phoenix—the mystical bird of immortality—each member, out of the fire of consummate love, renews his and her faith and joy for life. We see emerging from the entwining spirals of each birth three unique individuals who represent the unity of life that is found within the trinity. The parents' lives continue to unfold as does their creation—the child. All three have been totally, irrevocably changed yet remain eternally interconnected by a thought that was conceived in love.

Through such a dynamic interchange, humankind infinitely evolves—infinitely aspires to *absolute love*. Humankind's movement is wave-like. There is both an inward, contracting movement towards a more personal reality and an outer fluid motion towards the community of collective consciousness. As our perceptions become less dense, we become more free to respond to both these inner and outer worlds, the personal and the impersonal, the form and the formless, the earth and the heavens that nourish us. We become more aware at each turn of the spiral of life: of where I came from, of who I am, of what I am here for, and to where I shall be going. In a sense, we are continually evolving the resilience that is needed to adapt to our ever-changing environment.

"The sting" of this creative process is the law of impermanence. To create, to transform, is to be in a constant state of accepting new conditions, new contracts, new risks, new deaths, and finally, new realities. Life may not be easy, but it offers the potential of newness in the nowness.

However, nothing is lost in the act of acceptance and trust. Each new creation, each new thought, each new belief and action adds to the evolving Universe and to the continuing unfoldment of Life, *A Shared Creation*. Subsequent generations will find the unanswered questions of our time more easily answered and therefore will be drawn to ask questions that have not yet been conceived. If they are true seekers, they will hear a familiar voice, as ageless as time, say, "If I knew the answer, I would not need you." This is the collective, eternal voice of all preceding generations.

The King James' Version of God's name is "I AM THAT I AM." God is Love. Love as life is a shared creation that evolves through repeated struggle and resolution. Love, like energy, is a constant that cannot be created or destroyed but Love can evolve. Humankind is the variable of change within this orderly fixed universe. Perhaps the name of humankind is "I AM THAT I WILL BE." The ultimate joy will come with the complete understanding that we are both individually and collectively "The Conductors" and "The Transformers" found within God. Humankind has been given the unique gift of receiving and then transforming, through the life experience, knowledge into understanding, and thought into action and, thereby, formless Love into manifest Love.

We are co-creators in an evolving Collective Creative Consciousness called God.

Our life and our creations are God made visible.

To accept the totality of our humanness is to accept the totality of our Godliness.

Conception, birth and death are momentous events along life's continuum. The stages of pregnancy are stages of life. They point, as does life, to the path of personal transformation and collective unfoldment. Every step along the path of life is pregnant. Each stepping stone is a point in time, while the space that interconnects these stones is filled by our personal choices and so gives that path a special uniqueness. The silent space between the steps of life's path is the present moment, the music, while the stones are the beat. We are not who we think we are or what has been bequeathed for we are the instruments of Love itself. Our purpose is to make harmony out of life and to play with the symphony of the spheres the scores that are composed by Love. And, so, we are co-creators in the magnificent music of life which vibrates to all the shared sensate rhythms of the universe. Allow yourselves to be touched and to be played and so to resonate in life with Love.

The *Old Testament* is symbolic of a humanity that learned to serve by partaking of the tree of knowledge, comparison. The *New Testament* is symbolic of the immaculate conception (a child conceived free of parental projections) who chose the tree of everlasting life, a life without comparison and so learned of the spirit of interconnectedness. The *Third Testament* does not need to be written; the *Third Testament* only needs to be lived. The *Third Testament* is now and is the birth of immaculate conceptions into a singular community of service that is free of societal projections. In such a living context, the individual and humanity unfold simultaneously without the need to crucify or be crucified.

There is only a now and a beginning. Birth is found within oneself when the disharmony of differences are resolved in the spirit of total acceptance, and so transmuted to Love. Such acceptance of our humanness precludes the need for forgiveness or the judgment of guilt or blame. LOVE has no opposites and balance has no comparison. With this wisdom, we will know that we are a vital part of the evolving transformation of life and of Love. At that time, all of humanity will honor that we are indeed *A Gift from Love, A Gift of Life, A Shared Creation for All.*

A time will soon come in human evolution when we will no longer need the temporary experience of this earthly basinette. The fuel of conditional Love that is needed to maintain "Spaceship Earth" will have been transformed to the critical mass of unconditional Love that is needed to make the next journey possible.

And on that day of total trust the Creator and the Creations will rest as one. The work will have been done on earth as it was in heaven . . . and so it was good.

DAY EIGHT

. . . Love, like life, is pregnant and, as the thousand-petaled lotus, continues to unfold. There is no final octave in our evolutionary process. We are now approaching a new quantum of consciousness. Humanity has been preparing since creation for this next level of transformation. The hourglass is poised and waits to be turned over but once again. The last grains of sand will now be first to begin the next journey through the dark, narrow vortex into an existence of *Everlasting Light* . . . and so it was good.

DAY NINE

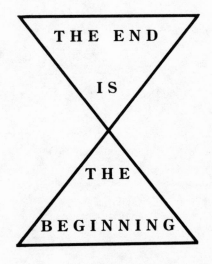

THE END IS THE BEGINNING

∞

Your Essence
is
Love
Your purpose
is
to evolve Love
Your Gift to Life
is
A Shared Creation
with Love

Paul

May 21, 1981

Bibliography

Baba Ram Dass. *Be Here Now.* New York: Crown Publishing, 1071.

Bach, Richards. *Illusions: The Adventures of a Reluctant Messiah.* New York: Delacorte Press, 1977.

Benson, Herbert. *The Relaxation Response.* New York: Avon, August, 1976.

Bentov, Itzhak. *Stalking The Wild Pendulum: On the Mechanics of Consciousness.* New York: E. P. Dutton, 1977.

Bing, Elizabeth, Marjorie. *Moving Through Pregnancy.* New York: Bantam Press, 1976.

Brenner, Paul. *Health Is A Question Of Balance.* New York: DeVorss Publishers, Marina Del Rey, CA.

_____. *The Impact of Pregnancy On Marriage: Medical Aspects of Human Sexuality.* July, 1977.

_____. *The Newborn's Impact on Parent's Marital and Sexual Relationship: Medical Aspects of Human Sexuality.* August, 1977.

Brown, Barbara. *New Mind, New Body.* New York: Harper and Row, 1974.

Buber, Martin. *Good and Evil.* New York: Charles Scribner's Sons, 1952, 1953.

_____. *I and Thou.* New York: Charles Scribner's Sons, 1958.

Capra, Fritjof. *The Tao of Physics.* Berkeley, Calif. Shambhala

Castaneda, Carlos. *A Separate Reality: Further Conversations With Don Juan.* New York: Simon & Schuster, May 1971.

_____. *Tales of Power.* New York: Simon & Schuster, 1974.

Chabon, Irwin. *Awake and Aware.* New York: Delacorte Press, 1969.

Cheek, David B. Maladjustment Patterns Apparently Related to Imprinting at Birth. *The American Journal of Clinical Hypnosis.* Vol. 18, Number 2, 2000 Van Ness Avenue, San Francisco, Calif., 94109, October, 1975.

_____. Sequential Head and Shoulder Movements Appearing with Age-Regression in Hyponosis to Birth. *The American Journal of Hypnosis,* Vol. 16, Number 4, San Francisco, Calif., April 1974.

Clark, Ronald W. *The Life and Times of Einstein.* New York: World Publishing Co., 1971.

Cummings, E. E. You Shall Above All Things Be Glad and Young. *The New Pocket Anthology of American Verse.* Ed. by Oscar Williams. Pocket Books, Wadington Square Press, 1972.

De Chardin, Pierre Teilhard. *Hymn of the Universe.* New York and Evanston: Harper Colophon Books, Harper & Row, 1965.

De Martino, Richard. Zen Buddhism and Psychoanalysis. *The Human Situation and Zen Buddhism.* New York: Colophon Books, Harper & Row, 1970.

Dewey, Jackie. *Of Life and Breath—A Holistic Approach* Beta Books, San Diego, CA.

Doman, Glenn. *What To Do About Your Brain Injured Child.* Doubleday, 1974.

Durden-Smith, Jo. *A Chemical Cure For Madness?* Terry Christian and the Startling Possibilities of DMT: Publication by the Ambassador International Cultural Foundation, Quest/May/June 1978, Vol. 2, Number 3, Pasadena, Calif.

Eaton, Evelyn. *I Send A Voice.* Wheaton, IL: Quest Book, Theosophical Publishing House, 1978.

Eccles, J. D. The Neurophysiological Basis of the Mind. *The Principles of Neurophysiological.* Oxford Clarendon Press, 1953.

_____. Possible Synoptic Mechanism Subserving Learning. Ed. by Karazman and Eccles. *Brain and Human Behavior,* 1972.

Engel, George. "The Clinical Application of The Biopsychosocial Model." *The American Journal of Psychiatry,* 137. May, 1980.

Franck, Frederick. *The Zen of Seeing: Seeing/Drawing as Meditation.* New York: Random House, 1973.

Frankl, Viktor E., *Man's Search For Meaning: An Introduction to Logotherapy.* New York: Simon & Schuster, 1963.

Freud, S. *The Interpretation of Dreams 1900* (Standard Ed.). London: Hogarth Press, 1953.

Fromm, Erich. Zen Buddhism and Psychoanalysis. New York: Harper Colophon Books, Harper & Row, 1970.

Gaskin, Ida May. *Spiritual Midwifery.* Summertown, Tennesee: Book Publishing Co., 1978.

Gibran, Kahlil. *The Prophet.* New York: Alfred A. Knopf, September, 1923.

Golas, Thaddeus. *The Lazy Man's Guide to Enlightenment,* Palo Alto, Calif. June, 1972.

Greenberg, Martin. *The Impact of Pregnancy on Marriage: Medical Aspects of Human Sexuality.* July, 1977.

_____. *The Newborn's Impact on Parent's Marital and Sexual Relationship: Medical Aspects of Human Sexuality.* August, 1977.

Grof, Stanislav. *Realms of Human Unconsciousness.* New York: Viking Press, 1977.

Halevi, Z'ev ben Shimon. *A Kabbalistic Universe.* New York; Samuel Weiser, 1977.

_____. *Adam and the Kabbalistic Tree.* New York: Samuel Weiser, 1974.

_____. *The Way of Kabbalah*. New York: Samuel Weiser, 1976.

Hammerstein, Oscar. Lyrics to Carrousel.

Hixon, Lex. *Coming Home*. New York: Doubleday, Anchor Press, 1978.

Israel, Leon and Isadore, Rubin. Sexual Relations During Pregnancy and the Post-Delivery Period. *Journal of Sex Information and Education Council of the U.S., Study Guide No. ; 1967.*

Janov, Arthur. *The Primal Scream*. Dell Press, 1972.

_____. *The Feeling Child*. Touchstone Books, 1975.

Joy, Brugh. *Joy's Way*. Los Angeles: J. Tarcher Publishers, 1979.

Jung, C. G. *Modern Man in Search of a Soul*. New York: Harvest Books.

Kubler-Ross, Elizabeth. *On Death and Dying*. New York: Macmillan Co., 1970.

Lamaze, F. *Painless Childbirth*. Henry Pegnery Co., Paris, 1970.

Lashley, K. S. *In Search of the Engram*. Symposium Soc Exp Biol, pp.454-482, 1950.

Leboyer, Frederick. *Birth Without Violence*. New York: Knopf, 1975.

_____. *Loving Hands*. New York: Knopf, 1976.

Levi, *The Aquarian Gospel of Jesus the Christ: The Philosophic and Practical Basis of the Religion of the Aquarian Age of the World.* Marina Del Rey, Calif., DeVorss & Co., 1972.

Levine, J. D., Gordon, N. C., Fields, H. L. "Placebo Effect," *The Lancet,* il. 654, 1978.

Liedenberg, B. *Expectant Fathers*. Paper given at the Annual Meeting of the American Orthopsychiatric Association in Washington, D.C., March 1967.

Lilly, John C. *The Centre of the Cyclone*. Bungay, Suffolk: The Chaucer Press, 1973.

Livingston, Robert. *Sensory Processing, Perception, and Behavior: Biological Foundation of Psychiatry*. Grenelland and Babay (Eds.). New York: Raven Press, 1976.

Lorenz, K. "Imprinting." *Journal Of Ornithology,* 83, 137, 1935.

McLoughlin, William. *Revivals, Awakenings, and Reform.* Chicago: University of Chicago Press, 1978.

Maltz, Maxwell. *Psycho-Cybernetics. A New Way to Get More Living Out of Life.* New York: Pocket Books, May 1969.

Masters, W. H., and Johnson, V. E. *Human Sexual Response. Boston: Little, Brown and Company, Ch. 10, 1966.*

May, Rollo. *The Courage to Create.* New York: Bantam Books, 1976.

Meyerowitz, J. H., and Feldman, H. "Transition to Parenthood." Psychiatric Research Report 20, pp.78-84. American Psychiatric Association, February 1966.

Montagu, Ashley. *Touching: The Human Significance of the Skin.* New York and London: Columbia University Press, 1971.

Moody, Raymond. *Reflections of Life After Life.* Bantam, 1978.

Moustakas, Clark. *Loneliness and Love.* Prentice-Hall, New York, 1972.

Namikoshi, Tokujiro. Japanese Finger-Pressure Therapy. Japan. Japan Publications, 1972.

Neilhardt, John G. *Black Elk Speaks: The Legendary "Book of Visions" Of An American Indian.* New York: Pocket Books, 1972.

Orr, Leanard, and Sondra Ray. *Rebirthing in the New Age.* 231 Adrian Road, Millbrae, Calif., Celestial Arts, 1977.

Ouspensky, P. D. *In Search of the Miraculous.* New York: Harcourt, Brace & World, 1949.

Oyle, Irving. *The Healing Mind.* New York: Pocket Books, 1976.

Panshin, Alexei. *The Thurb Revolution.* New York: Grosset and Dunlap.

_____ and Morris, N. "Engrossment." *American Journal of Orthopsychiatry,* (44)(4):520, 1974.

Pelletier, Kenneth R. *Mind As Healer, Mind As Slayer.* New York: Delacourte Press, 1977.

Progoff, Ira. *A Journal Workshop.* New York: Dialogue House Library, 1975.

_____. *Jung, Synchronicity, and Human Destiny.* New York: Dell Publishing Co., March, 1975.

Reed, Grantley. *Childbirth Without Fear.* New York: Harper & Row, 1972.

Rilke, Rainer, Maria. *Letters To A Young Poet.* Translation by M. D. Herter Norton, New York: W. W. Norton, 1954.

_____. *Poems From The Book Of Hours.* New York: New Directions Paperbook, 1975.

Russell, Bertrand. *The ABC Of Relativity.* New York: Mentor Books.

Saint Augustine. "Confessions." Translated and annotated by J. G. Pelkington, M.A., New York. International Collector's Library American Headquarters.

Scholem, Gershom. *Kabbalah.* Jerusalem, Israel: Keter Publishing House, 1977.

_____. *Zohar, The Book of Splendor: Basic Readings From The Kabbalah.* New York: Schocken Books, 1963.

Segal, S. J. (Ed.). *Imagery: Current Cognitive Approach.* Academic Press, 1971.

Serrano, Miguel. *C. G. Jung and Hermann Hesse.* New York: Schocken Books, 1966.

Spalding, D. A., "On Instinct." *Macmillan's Magazine,* Feb. 1873, 287, 289 (Quotations from James, W. Principles of Psychology, 1890, Henry Holt, V.II, p.396).

Suzuki, D. T. "Zen Buddhism and Psychoanalysis," Lectures on Zen Buddhism. New York: Colophon Books, Harper & Row, 1970.

Suzuki, Shunryu. "Zen Mind, Beginner's Mind." Informal talks on Zen Meditation and Practice. New York: Tokyo: Weatherhill, 1970.

Taub, Edward. "The Telling of A Story," submitted to *American Journal of Pediatrics.*

Teilhard de Chardin, Pierre. *The Phenomenon of Man.* New York: Harper and Row.

_____. *Hymn of the Universe.* New York: Harper and Row.

Tillich, Paul. *The Courage To Be.* Yale University Press, New Haven and London, 1979.

Tinbergen, Hikolaas. "Ethology and Stress Diseases." Lecture delivered in Stockholm, Sweden, December 1973. Published with permission of the Nobel Foundation, 1974.

Tinning, Adele Gerard. *God's Way of Life.* February 1971, 3650 Mississippi Street, San Diego, Calif., 92104.

Trethowan, W. H., and Conlon, M.F. "The Couvade Syndrome." *British Journal of Psychiatry,* March 1965.

Underhill, Evelyn. *Mysticism. A Study in the Nature and Development of Man's Spiritual Consciousness.* New York: E. P. Dutton.

Watson, Burton. *The Complete Works of Chuang Tzu.* Columbia University Press, 1970.

White, T.H. *The Book of Merlyn.* University of Texas Press, Austin and London.

Whitman, Walt. *Poems of Walt Whitman.* New York: Thomas Y. Crowell Co., Apollo Edition, 1971.

Winfree, Arthur. "Resetting Biological Clocks." *Physics Today,* March 1975.

Zeeman, E. "Catastrophy Theory." *Scientific American,* April, 1976.

The Holy Bible—Revised Standard Version. Thomas Nelson & Sons: New York: 1952.

The I Ching. Bollingen Series XIX. New Jersey: Princeton University Press, 1975.

The Kybalion, by Three Initiates (No Author). The Yogi Publication Society, Chicago (out-of-print).